my life in a Tutu

JACKIE MADDEN HAUGH

Published in the United States by WriteLife Publishing
(An imprint of Boutique of Quality Books Publishing Company)
www.writelife.com

Printed in the United States of America
978-1-939371-74-4 (p)
978-1-939371-75-1 (e)
Library of Congress Control Number: 2015930495

Book design by Robin Krauss, www.lindendesign.biz
Cover design by David Grauel, www.davidgrauel.com

Also by Jackie Madden Haugh

75 Beats to a Happy Heart
Fall 2014

Upcoming Books in the Tutu Series:

Tipsy in a Tutu

The Promise I Kept

Dedication

This book is dedicated to my four children, Michelle, Jenni, Lauren, and Tim, who were patient with their mother as she struggled to find her voice.

Living for nearly fifty years with my thoughts, dreams, and opinions guarded under lock and key, I was often afraid to speak my own truth. Insecurity and low self-esteem seemed to scream that what I had to impart on any given subject—even if it was the story of my life—would be found irrelevant. But as I took the journey to self-discovery through the written word, my children anxiously waited for the finished product, for they never doubted in my abilities, even if I at times lost sight.

We all need a champion from time to time who believes in us, that relentless cheerleader always pushing us toward victory. I am fortunate that I found my advocate in the hearts of my kids.

Prologue

After a three-year separation in 2004, my painful divorce from a twenty-two year marriage was final. My four children were beginning to blow the Haugh family popsicle stand for college, and I was redefining my life as a divorcee.

"Oh my God, Jackie, you have to write a book!" my dear friend Libby told me after I finished relating my latest escapade as a single woman at a cocktail party.

"Yeah right, Lib. Like I'm going to write a book!" Looking into her encouraging eyes, I wondered how she could even think such a thing.

"Who'd want to read about me?" I asked incredulously.

"Your kids would." She smiled, her ebony eyes dancing at the idea.

At first, I found the idea ridiculous. English was always my worst class in school. I could barely write a coherent sentence and was completely challenged in the comprehension department. Reading a book was an intimidating task that froze my mind and left me staring at the wall counting spiders. At least ridding my house of unwanted guests was productive and a lesson I knew how to attack. A swift bat with the back of the book would bring the subject to full closure.

Since I was ten, I'd suffered from a severe case of the "I'm not good enough" flu, that nasty little germ that silently wove its way into the psyche of many little girls in the 1960s. I was sure there was nothing extraordinary about me that was worth putting on paper. The effort would just lead to a waste of my precious time: time I could be spending going to singles parties and meeting other lonely, pathetic individuals just like me; time I could be lying on the couch watching reruns of *Law and Order SVU*; time I could be enjoying a lovely self-imposed pity party, with a fine glass of buttery Chardonnay.

But while driving home that evening, I reexamined whether such a project would be something my children would find worthwhile. In their eyes, I was just a mom. A woman who loved them unconditionally and who'd always be at the other end of the phone line when they called for help.

When I'd discovered my own mother's writings several years after her death, I found myself wishing I had read them while she was alive. It would have given me more insight into her as a woman, and not just a mother. Perhaps taking on this challenge would help my own children do the same. The humanness in all of us unfolds in a complicated process, but if it's in written form, we're able to sit back and reflect on it, rather than criticize, attack, or be confused.

As I read through pages and pages of her perfect penmanship, I discovered her impenetrable veneer had hidden a vast array of frailties that, on paper, were completely exposed. My mother in her youth was always a force to be reckoned with: strong, vibrant, and articulate. By comparison, in my mind I was just a dull copper penny person, tossed aside. She was that coveted newly minted, shining silver dollar.

But, there on the blue lines of her brown faded journal, insecurities screamed a tune I was all too familiar with: feelings of doubt and lack of self-worth. I pored over the lines that questioned her own self-worth, loves she once lost, and dreams unfulfilled. My eyes stung as tears found their way down my cheeks. If only I'd known this earlier in my life and seen her as human, perhaps it would have helped me be more patient with my own insecurities.

Reflecting on my life, I began to see it as a kind of drama, with me on center stage playing several different parts simultaneously. With each story line, I was a unique character as I ran to my dress-up box to find the perfect costume. In my youth, there was the mime in a brightly colored clown outfit and white painted face that had no voice and never spoke. Wearing my blue-and-green-plaid uniform, I was the Catholic schoolgirl searching for an ambiguous thing called faith. In dirty overalls, I became the warden of a wild animal park trying to keep her children in their cages and out of harm's way. Among other characters was a nurse who cared for the sick and dying, the little girl longing for the fairy tale of Happily Ever After, and a ballerina who pranced through it all while desperately trying to stay balanced and on her toes.

I often wanted to hold others responsible for the limitations some roles imposed. It's so much easier to stand up straight when life's constraints are caused by someone else.

Blaming my mother for always trying to control the things I did—from how I wore my hair and makeup to the way I represented the family when I stepped outside of the Madden home—was a great cop-out for not allowing myself to be adventurous.

I accused my former husband of emotionally and physically abandoning me once his dynasty became teenagers. The world beyond our front door was far more exciting than his dull, exhausted wife lying on the couch after a long day of driving four kids to all their afterschool activities and dealing with hormonal explosions.

And I resented my brothers for being such a strong force of nature that they had gotten the lion's share of my parents' attention. It would be years until I realized I had played a major role in my past and how my life turned out.

The two-year journey it took to complete this work became an important part of my own healing and self-discovery.

From the time I was a little thing, I only knew myself as the good girl, that people pleaser who wanted everyone happy, even if it came at my expense. Constantly forsaking my opinions and desires, I lived in the dark, not knowing what I was capable of, let alone who I was. Then, at fifty years old, my divorce ripped what little solid foundation I did have out from under me. By being brutally honest with myself and taking responsibility for my part in my life, I was finally able to swim free from that ocean of broken dreams I once frantically treaded water in.

The journey also brought an awareness that led me down a new path, to the spiritual connection with God that I was missing. Through it all, I realized a better understanding of my place in the world, my motives for the things I do, and my connection to those I love.

My mother always told me it was never too late for more soul searching, that we were constant students in the classroom of life. As she lay in the hospital toward the end, we had countless discussions about her life, what she was proud of, and where she felt she had failed.

"Jackie, we are forever a work in progress," she said, as her feeble and infirm hand held mine. "By soul searching and delving deep into our thoughts and dreams, we never stop growing. We're done only when we make that final journey home."

If I were to leave one pearl of wisdom to my children, it would be to never lose sight of who they are, away from the external labels that we place on ourselves. Looks, power, wealth, fame, and relationships are mere garments, costumes that need to be worn lightly, because they can disappear in a heartbeat. It's not the jobs we do or the material items we possess that define us as human beings. We can find who we are by simply looking into our souls, listening to our hearts, and discovering how well we rise after falling.

Now when I have a new character to portray, I no longer run to the dress-up box to don a costume that will mask my feelings and help me survive. Instead, I pick out the most flamboyant outfit I can find to accentuate my mood and celebrate the moment. The biggest mistake in life is not taking the time to live.

Isadora Duncan

At eight years old, I was expelled from Miss Nancy's School of Dance. I was on track to be the perfect little girl, but for one brief moment in my young life, I rebelled. Sure, I'd done naughty things, like stick my finger into the softened butter on our kitchen table, then dip it into the sugar bowl for a tasty treat. Or lie that it wasn't me who stole the money from Dad's dresser drawer. But this moment was my one and only act of true childhood mutiny.

From the second I was born, my mother, Lassie Pearce Madden, had been preparing me for that auspicious day when she'd enroll me in my first ballet class. Groomed to be a prima ballerina herself, she loved the world of dance but gave up pursuing her own craft after junior high school.

"I was being trained to be a star," she once said reflectively. "But my teacher was so mean and whipped my legs when I didn't stand straight enough. I decided to quit. How I wish I'd stayed with it."

Owning her mistake in her late thirties, she knew it was too late for her. That swan song had exited stage left long ago. After that, my mom wallowed in the world of *has been*. But her daughter was just beginning to blossom. She decided I should pick up where she'd left off. Unfortunately, there was just one problem. She was the only one feeling the excitement.

"Okay, honey, this is going to be so much fun!" Mom was chirping like a sparrow welcoming the first suggestion of spring in the air. Putting her favorite album, *The Nutcracker,* on the record player, she turned up the volume to "Dance of the Sugar Plum Fairy" and twirled me in circles. "Stand on your tippy-toes, Jackie. Keep your tummy in tight. Dancers never slouch."

Before I learned to read, my first picture books were old family photo albums where Mom relived cherished moments over and over with me on her lap.

"These are my dolls. There is your Great Aunt Esther, Grammy, and Grandpa. Oh! That is our dog," she repeated tirelessly, like a recording.

I'd looked at those pictures so many times, I could almost hear in my mind what was coming next.

"And this is me in my ballerina outfit. I was on toe at a very early age." Wistfully, Mom ran her fingers over the faded sepia images as endearing memories took her back in time.

On the delicate, tissue-thin pages before me was a frightening black-and-white image of my mother in her knee-length limp tutu with a scooped neckline embellished with billowing silk organza ruffles, looking more like ten yards of fabric drawn together into a ruff (the thick neckwear worn in Western Europe in the 1600s). But instead of choking the neckline, the fabric was drooping off her shoulders. On her long, skinny legs, satin laces wove back and forth from tiny pink shoes tied just below her bony knees. In my mind, all this was creepy enough. Weren't ballerinas supposed to look like elegant swans in pretty, short tutus and black, tight-fitting leotards (with a few diamonds on them)? But it was what they'd stuck on her head that made me quiver.

"Mommy, why are you wearing weeds in your hair?"

"Weeds? Those aren't weeds." Mom studied the image, puzzled. "That's my tiara. Don't I look pretty?"

A wreath of garden flowers sat low on her wide forehead. It looked more like a crown of fist-sized brittle clumps of tumbleweeds, just waiting for the first strong wind to take them wandering. Fortunately, they were held in place with a thin black velvet ribbon. I wondered if the painful expression on her face was due to what appeared to be thorns intertwined in the headpiece or the fact that she had been standing on her toes for too long.

"Will I have to wear something like that to dance?" I asked, trembling at the thought.

It wasn't that I minded being in costume. From the time I was old enough to dress myself, I'd loved wearing strange outfits and pretending to be any character I wanted during the process of putting on the final costuming touches. But, unlike my mother—who always looked like a movie star straight from the pages of *Vogue* magazine—my end product was typically unconventional and eclectic. Instead of emulating the traditional ballerina in her cotton candy–colored ensemble, with precise, technically correct moves, my style resembled that of Isadora Duncan, the creator of modern dance in the late 1800s.

On a cold, rainy Saturday afternoon near my fifth birthday, my mother and I had watched an old black-and-white movie about Duncan's life. Enamored with her style, I wanted to know who she was.

"Mommy, who is that lady?" I asked, watching her float across the screen.

"Just some nutty woman who thinks she can dance."

"Wow," I whispered, mesmerized by Duncan's dancing. "I like the way she moves."

"That is *not* dancing," my mother mumbled, acting disgusted at the vision.

How could my mom not like this style of dance? I was in awe of this flamboyant creature and wanted to re-create her sense of fashion. It was obvious she felt free: hair wild and blowing in the wind as she twirled her body, barefoot with rainbow-colored scarves streaming off her neck and shoulders.

To re-create her style, I began to wear unrestrictive, multicolored skirts and long shawls from the dress-up box. With rows and rows of brightly colored beaded necklaces around my short neck, and gold bangles traveling up both arms, I pranced around our house free and unfettered, waving my limbs in abandon.

That's what I was doing the day Mom came to get me ready for my first ballet class.

"Honey, take all that stuff off and come see what I bought you. You're going to look so sweet."

There on my bed, laid out in order of application for my bubble-shaped body, was the beginning of a tortured two-year career as a tiny dancer. At the end were pink ballet shoes, funny little slippers with a strap across the top, and elastic strings that would prove to never stay tied. Next were the customary pink tights that gravity would constantly pull south from my blubbery midsection, leaving a rumple just below my bottom. This not only looked odd, but also created much discomfort.

"Mom, I look like I'm still wearing diapers," I yelled, trying to pull the tight spandex back up again.

"Oh, honey. It doesn't look that bad. Maybe I can buy you another pair in a larger size. I want you comfy."

No! I wanted to scream. To me, comfy was being in my play clothes, sitting in the sandbox or climbing a tree.

Topping off the costume was a lackluster black leotard, which did nothing to complement my out-of-proportion physique.

Where are the frills, ribbon, or lace? I wanted to cry. *This is boring.*

"Now, let's get dressed. You're going to look so cute," Mom said in her singsongy way, as she led me to the garments. "Once we get this on, I'll put your hair in a bun."

"A bun! No, Mommy, not a bun," I pleaded. "You always pull my hair too tight."

Exasperated at my fuss, she turned and forcefully tried to make me believe: *this will be fun.*

An hour later, my body stuffed into spandex and my hair glued to the sides of my head, I stood in a dark school auditorium with twenty other squirming kindergartners. We wrapped our small hands around a makeshift ballet barre, tummies sucked in tight and feet in first position, as we desperately tried to create the perfect plié without falling over.

"Jackie, stand up straight. Hold in your stomach," Miss Nancy ordered. "And stop wiggling. What's wrong with you?"

"Excuse me, what time do I get to go home?" I asked, carefully raising my hand straight to the ceiling.

"Why? Aren't you having fun?" Miss Nancy asked sharply.

There was that word *fun* again.

Week after week, as I suffered through the hell of ballet lessons, I became less coordinated and extremely disruptive. Flexible I was not, and as each girl fell easily into the splits, I had to find ways to divert attention away from my ineptitude.

"Hey Paula, watch this," I snickered, hanging upside down off the barre. With my right knee cocked over the wooden pole, I dangled my head and arms toward the floor. "I bet you can't do this."

"Jackie!" Miss Nancy screamed. "What are you doing?"

"Sorry." I quickly reassembled myself to try to act like the other clones in black.

When it came time to practice our moves across the floor, instead of placing my arms in the required controlled position, I flailed them in the air as if I were trying to catch a hummingbird darting from one flower's nectar to another.

"Jackie, if you don't stop fooling around, I'm going to call your mother!" Miss Nancy threatened.

I knew how uncomfortable my life at home would be if my mother was caught off guard by a call about any misconduct in school. Having a learning disability that went undiagnosed, my attention span and desire for learning were never my strong suit. Consequently, every Tuesday I found myself in detention for out-of-control whispering.

"Don't call her. I'll be good. I promise."

Later that afternoon, with my face glued to the television, I heard the telephone ring. The tone of my mom's voice was unlike any I'd heard before. All of a sudden, I realized who it was.

Oh no! It's Miss Nancy. With super speed, I made a dash for my secret hiding place, the dark cave under my bed.

"What?" I heard Mom say in a mortified voice. "What do you mean, you think Jackie's not meant to dance? How ridiculous! She is going to be a great dancer."

On the other end of the phone, my annoying prune of a teacher evidently tried to explain why I was not welcome in class anymore. I could only imagine what she must be saying: "Mrs. Madden, Jackie just doesn't have it. She's clumsy and awkward, plus her tummy won't fit into the costumes. What do you feed her?"

"My daughter is perfect. I don't know what you are talking about," Mom hissed.

"On top of her not being in shape to dance, she's a behavior problem. We just can't deal with her anymore." It would be just like Miss Nancy to add, "Maybe baton twirling would be a good activity. She seems to like to throw things. Better yet, how about football? She definitely has the body for it."

Exposed at last, there I was, a disgrace to the family name. No one on either side of my parents' long lineage had ever been expelled or kicked out of anything. Seeing the wounded look on my mother's face and the disappointment in her eyes that afternoon, as she folded up my ballet outfit and placed it in the garage with the other discarded items that were no longer needed, I first cried knowing I'd hurt her. But then I made a vow to myself.

I'm going to show everyone I can dance.

No professional was ever going to tell me again I couldn't do something because I didn't fit the mold. I may not have been right for Miss Nancy, but I was born to dance. I could feel it in my soul.

Determined to perform in my own way, I chose to listen to the beat of my internal drummer as I practiced my own sense of style. This would give me years of immense personal enjoyment—with or without a partner.

Hmm, if I tie this rope to my door, I can pretend it's my dance partner and the cord is his arm, I speculated, getting ready to break loose with my invisible friend.

Music blaring from my pink plastic AM radio, I rolled my body in toward the door as the rope encircled my waist, and, then with complete lack of inhibition, back out again. Lifting it up in the air, I twirled underneath, ending in a back bend. And for the finale, a backward somersault. Flipping my legs over my head, I jumped up to start all over again.

See! I can dance.

During those formative years, I learned to jitterbug, boogie, plus bump and grind with the wooden gate to my secret world. Every Saturday morning, staking a claim on the family television set to watch *American Bandstand*, I took copious mental notes as I studied each move. At the end of the show, back to my room I'd go to practice in front of my full-length mirror what I'd seen. By the time I was a teenager, I was an accomplished performer at the local teen club dances. Every Friday night, one of the local parishes hosted a mixer for all the Catholic teenagers to attend. I became the envy of all my friends in high school, as I twirled circles around any partner. I even made gangly, pimple-faced sixteen-year-old boys look like superstars.

"Now stand there and don't move," I'd whisper, dragging the next unsuspecting victim to the center of the room. "Just turn when I tell you to turn and I'll do the rest. You'll be fine."

This determination to never again be told how to do something taught me that self-rule would be the key to any success I'd achieve. Whether it was my grades or a job, I was going to make it in my own way, without assistance from anyone else. I dug my Capricorn heels firmly into the shag carpet, and Stubborn became my middle name when taking care of my business.

Years later, at the age of thirty-eight, a miraculous event occurred.

I'd received my Health and Fitness certificate from our local YMCA. With that knowledge, I developed an exercise program for my son's kindergarten class, composed of dance movements intermixed with games to children's music. In May 1994, Sioux Lehner, the director of a local studio, *Dance Attack*, witnessed my creation at the end-of-the-year talent show.

There on stage, fifty kindergarten-age students, dressed in green with Tyrannosaurus Rex headpieces tied firmly under their tiny chins, did a silly break dance number to "Dino the Dinosaur," bringing the house down in tears of laughter.

Sioux came racing up to catch me afterward. She offered me a wild idea.

"How would you like to teach dance to my baby classes?"

Stunned, I stared blankly back at her. But the thought of flitting around the dance studio with a bunch of three-year-olds made me giggle. It also terrified me.

"Sioux, I have no formal education," I responded, surprised she would even suggest such a thing. "I can't do that."

"You don't need any. All you need is a love of children and a little rhythm. The rest will come together. Look at what you put together tonight *without* training. I'll teach you!"

To my delight, I found that Sioux and I had the same philosophy when it came to creating joy to music. Unlike Miss Nancy, who was rigid and nasty, Sioux allowed me the freedom to teach the way I knew best: with a lot of love and humor.

The children and I were perfect for each other and developed a mutual admiration society. I adored those precious three- and four-year-olds, and they in turn delighted in my style.

Using props from my children's dress-up box at home, we pranced and spun around the room, pretending to be fairy princesses or their favorite animals. While I knew they were required to learn certain steps, I focused on what I enjoyed best about dance: the expression on the children's faces, not the perfection in their bodies. The children and I may have had little talent, but we sure were cute.

In contrast to Miss Nancy's shows, which were dull and monotonous, with music dating back to my grandmother's era, *Dance Attack* productions were spectacular. It was in this studio that I experienced my first Ziegfeld Follies stage-like experience with larger-than-life props, bright lights, and glitzy apparel for the children and myself.

"Jackie, what the hell are you wearing?" I heard a friend ask at the end-of-the-year recital.

Looking at the mounds of fabric billowing off my body, I replied confidently, "My costume. Why? What's wrong with it?"

Our number was centered on a maypole. Twenty-five preschoolers and I wore outfits that resembled the traditional Swiss attire worn on national holidays. Brightly colored bodices hoisted sleeves just off the shoulders, and multicolored ribbons crisscrossed our chests. The tulle slips consisted of five layers of netting that poofed the top skirt out to the sides, making me look like I was wearing an open umbrella. It was the perfect shield for all the kids to hide under, should there be a water leak from the overhead fire extinguishers on stage. I had a crown of garden flowers in my hair and pink ballet shoes with ribbons crisscrossing my not-so-slender legs.

My friend was correct. I looked ridiculous.

"Oh my God, Jackie, I wouldn't be caught dead in that," she laughed. "You must really love those kids to wear that in public."

For a moment, I was almost offended. Even though my friend was being snarky, she was correct about the love part. There was no way I was going to allow those babies on stage without me. And if my Swedish ballerina outfit made me look ludicrous, then so be it.

"Yes, I do love those kids." I smiled back. "And if they have to be out there in these God-awful things, then I'm right there with them."

Despite the fact that some children turned left when everyone else was going right, and a few got tangled in the ribbons of the pole, the performance was a success. We were definitely not the most accomplished group of the show. But we were the showstopper of the evening because of twenty-five proud, smiling, and happy children waving at their mommies and daddies. Blowing kisses, they took their bows and skipped merrily off the stage.

"Jackie, I think they loved us," four-year-old Hailey screeched with joy, as I pulled her back behind the curtain. "We must be really good!"

Giggling over the fact that we were far from good (in fact, it was total chaos), I marveled at how well behaved the children were. Thinking back to my first recitals, I recalled my face peering through a cardboard daisy, petals sticking out in every direction, and looking miserable. On stage, if the slightest thing went wrong, we never heard the end of it from Miss Nancy. Not only would we get a tongue-lashing, but we would be instructed to do one hundred push-ups the following class. No wonder I had hated it.

This delightful moment reinforced my lifelong belief that dance should always begin with a smile on the face, a twinkle in the eye, and the communication it brings to the heart before it ever connects with the feet.

For me, when we allow music to sing to the spirit, the heart is free to dance unencumbered, no matter what age we become.

This experience also made me realize this was how I wanted my life to be. For thirty-eight years, I'd struggled to live a perfect life, to please others, putting their needs above my own at every turn. Unfortunately, all that ever did was leave me feeling frustrated and empty. No matter what I did or how hard I tried, it never seemed to be enough.

Walking off that stage that evening, I decided it was time to throw my self-imposed restricted life into the same box where that humdrum black leotard and those pink tights resided, and make decisions that pleased only me. It was a task I thought would be as easy as waving my childhood kaleidoscope silk shawl over my head.

What I wasn't prepared for was that it would take another twelve years for me to even begin to accomplish it.

The Good Girl

The role of the *good girl* would be my Achilles heel for nearly fifty years, but when my mother passed away in 2003, so too did my burning desire to constantly please. Because of the deep love I felt for her, my never-ending need for her approval had become a bear trap I could not release myself from. On that sad day, I decided it was time to pull apart the iron claws of that lifelong snare. With that release, the monster within that prevented me from acknowledging it was okay to not live a perfect life, and occasionally be selfish, ran for the woods, never to be seen again. I was finally free to be me, whoever that was.

Smashed in the middle of my family's birth order, I lived in a world filled with testosterone, aggressive play, and loud noises. Life was bad enough with all the cars, baseballs, wrestling, and noise that came with two brothers, but when Michael was born, I was sure God was mad at me for disobeying my parents. I often found myself wondering: *How in the hell did I get into this family?* As far as I was concerned, it was cruel and unjust punishment to a little six-year-old girl. Couldn't I have had at least one sister?

To escape the noise in those early days of the 1950s, I spent most of my time locked away in the fantasy world of my bedroom. There my dolls and I created a world where everyone got along and, most importantly, everyone loved me. I was the center of my own universe. But on occasion, when I got lonely or bored, I wanted someone to play with. It usually happened right before the dinner hour.

"Davey, will you play with me?" I'd beg my older brother.

David, two years older and the heir apparent, was born an old soul. There was always order to his life and his playtime. Unfortunately, to him I was a pesky bug, constantly flying in his face, that couldn't be swatted away.

"Can I play?" I asked again, whining as I stood in the middle of his make-believe war. "I'll be whatever you want me to be."

"Jackie, go away!" he grunted, never looking up from his miniature toy soldiers.

"How about we play army? You and Tim can be soldiers, and I'll be the nurse?"

"Jackie, leave me alone!" David yelled, this time pushing me away from his medieval castle. "I don't want to play right now. You're bugging me."

"I know! Let's play baseball?" I tried again. "You'll be the pitcher, Tim can be the batter, and I can play left out." "That's left field, stupid."

"Okay, whatever." I continued to beg. "I promise I won't let any balls go by me."

"Jackie, get out of here or I'm calling Mom," David cried, frustrated. "Why do you always have to bug me when I want to be alone?"

Walking away, I dreamed of ways to get my big brother's attention. But, like the tiny men he had swimming in the moat after they'd been dumped off the castle wall, I had no idea what it would take for me to be allowed inside his fort.

With my other brother Tim I fared a little better. Twenty months younger than me, he was just as desperate as I for companionship, so we took turns doing what the other wanted.

"Let's play house," I suggested, heading for my well-equipped room, complete with doll-sized kitchen and table.

"No, I want to go to the creek and climb trees," Tim responded, bolting for the door.

Running after him, I grabbed his hand as it reached for the knob. "It's my turn to choose. You never want to play house anymore. I'm tired of doing what you want."

"Nope, I'm going outside." He grinned, shoving me aside.

Soon the scuffle began. Like puppies at play, we found ourselves rolling in circles on the floor. Only this time it became serious business. From out of nowhere, his dirty fingernails found their way across my face, leaving three deep scratches on my right cheek.

"Ouch!" I screamed. "You're gonna get it now."

While I may have been the most cooperative child in the Madden household, I definitely was no wuss. In an instant, my left hook landed in just the right spot, blood now gushing from his nose.

"Mom!" he wailed, running off to plug up the hole in the dike.

"Sorry, Tim," I whispered, a tremor in my voice, and ran to my favorite hiding place under my bed. There I slipped into the darkness where no one would find me. For years, it was my safe haven when things got heated in our home.

From 1950 to 1958, one baby after another descended on the Madden family home, four kids in all. It was a time of chaos that my mother quelled with her tight-ship schedule, and a lot of yelling.

"Damn it to hell, Tim," she screamed, chasing my brother through the house. "Get in your room!"

My brother's energy levels were at an all-time high. My mother not only needed, but demanded, order if she was to retain her sanity. The best way for her to achieve this was getting us all in bed at the same time.

"Mommy, look at me! I'm all ready for bed," I cried out, delighted as I ran from my room to show I had my pajamas on.

Brushing past me without looking, she darted after David to stop him from torturing his younger brother. "David, stop teasing Tim and go brush your teeth!"

"Mommy, I'm ready," I tried again.

Just like every night, no answer. Somehow, once again, I became invisible when I was doing what I was supposed to do.

My youngest brother, Michael, was whimpering as he toddled his way past the ruckus. Since he was the baby, my mom jumped at his slightest cry. Quickly, she scooped him up to protect him from the scuffle erupting on the living room floor.

"Mommy, I'm in the bathroom brushing my teeth," I mumbled with a mouthful of toothpaste.

Still no answer.

Bedtime in the Madden home was never the quiet ending to a lovely day. What started off as a dull rumble would crescendo to all-out warfare between the boys and my mother. As the shouting began, I found my way to my pillow, fearful that in the heat of the moment I might be mistaken for my brother Tim and get the spanking meant for him. Just like she sometimes mixed up our names when shouting in a fury, my mother's hand occasionally missed her intended target, landing on the one who got in the middle.

"Tim, get off the counter," Mom demanded, grabbing him out of the kitchen. "You may not have any cookies. It's bedtime."

"Tim, now what are you doing?" she yelled, as she came from putting Michael in his crib. "Turn off that water! It's running all over the bathroom floor."

No sooner would she get one son settled, than another would break loose from his chains and go wandering.

"Come here, Michael." She noticed he'd escaped his cage. "It's time for night-night."

The range of emotion was mind blowing. Her voice traveled from loving and sweet to a full-on crescendo of force.

"*Damn it, David!* Turn off the TV. I said it was time for bed."

"Mommy, I AM in bed." I tried one more time before attempting to fall asleep. *I'm being really good. Please see me!*

I wanted to be seen as a good girl and, in return, to be loved for it. Sadly, I felt unimportant compared to everyone else in my family. What I didn't comprehend in those early years was that it's easy to ignore the perfect child. She needs no attention because she's doing what's required.

But in our family, perfection didn't just mean how we acted. It was in the way we looked. That said to the world that the Madden family was special. That grooming began early, but for some reason, I received extra attention in how I looked before I left the family compound. Perhaps since I was the only girl, my mom felt I needed more instruction in the feminine department. But, as I struggled to find ways to fit in with my brothers, the one easy way to do that was to dress like them. Party dresses, unless we were actually going to a party, were not a fun daily occurrence.

In my mother's eyes, the Madden children were the most beautiful, precious, and flawless creatures God ever created. We were her finest achievement, and much of her identity was wrapped up in how we looked when we left the house. If an outsider praised us on our appearance, my mom took that as a reflection on her parenting. In her eyes, flawless children equaled a flawless mothering style.

"All right, kids, time to get ready for the day. I want you all looking your best." The morning drill would begin. "Make sure your shoes are clean and, boys, tuck in your shirts. Jackie, let's put you in a pretty dress."

"Can I wear play clothes?" I would ask carefully, but always knowing the real answer even at the tender age of four.

"No, honey. I'm taking you all to the matinee this afternoon."

"But the boys aren't dressed up," I would say carefully, for fear her demeanor might change to something less pleasant as a result of my nagging. I was probably the only little girl in town who was required to wear her Sunday best just to see a B-rated, black-and-white Roy Rogers western.

"Jackie, you know whenever you walk out that door you represent the family. Now let's find something cute."

Just as I was finishing pulling up the itchy nylon slip, Mom would call from the bathroom, "Jackie, come here and let me fix your hair. You look so adorable in two ponytails."

From the moment I had hair long enough to put into a rubber band, I wore two perfectly coiled Shirley Temple corkscrews on each side of my head. Over the years, much to my embarrassment, these twists of strawberry-blond hair grew longer and longer, until in fifth grade they fell down to my waist.

"Mom, do you think I could wear my hair down?" I periodically asked in moments of passing courage.

"Oh, baby, you look so much cuter and neater with your hair off your face." She took a moment from whatever she was doing to explain her reasoning. "I hear all the time how precious you are. Let's just leave your hair the way it is."

To continue pleasing her, I wore those wretched pigtails until I entered sixth grade. My friends were allowed to play with their looks beginning in second grade. How I longed to go to school with my hair down looking like I just climbed out of bed. Instead, I walked around with the hairdo of a three-year-old on a preteen head.

"Mom, all my friends are starting to cut their hair and wear it in a flip," I began quickly. It was 1964, and bouffant hairdos were becoming a thing of the past. Easy breezy hairstyles that took little time to manufacture were all the rage, and I was tired of all the pulling and gluing that went into constructing my coifed head. "You can buy these really cute bows and hook them on the sides of my head so hair won't fall over my eyes. What do you think?"

"Hmm, I don't know." Mom paused, frowning. "You may be sorry. Once it's gone, it takes forever to grow back."

"But my hair is beginning to fall out. I have holes on parts of my scalp because the rubber bands are too tight." I continued carefully, afraid she'd cut me off. "Don't you think it needs a rest? I really don't want to go bald." *Besides, I'm twelve years old, not two.*

After carefully looking at my scalp and eyeing the open patches of skin where hair once grew, she finally saw the light.

"Okay, honey," she sighed. "You're right. I don't want you looking like Yul Brynner." So, off we went for my first real haircut in an actual beauty parlor.

I was amazed at how much better everything smelled than in the barbershop where Mom took me to get my bangs trimmed at the same time the boys got their ears lowered. In the beauty parlor, small crystal bottles lined the counter of the hairdresser's station, and fragrances of lilac and spiced apple wafted around my head.

Even the conversation was different. All I ever heard in Frank's barbershop was discussion about the latest sporting event. But in Betty's Beauty Palace, stories were intermixed with snickers and sneers.

"Did you hear what Trudy's been doing with Gina's husband?" Ethel asked my mother.

"It's not nice to spread rumors. I don't want to hear about it," Mom sneered.

"Oh, Lassie. You're such a stick in the mud," Ethel giggled.

"I'd like to hear about it," I chimed in, knowing it must be juicy if my mother wouldn't talk about it in front of me.

"Jackie, it's none of your business. Just be quiet and let's get this over with."

And before Ethel could even begin her tale of smut, the ponytails were gone, and out the door I went ready to grow up.

During those formative preteen years, I became extremely self-reliant. Was it the new hairdo or the memory of my dance expulsion? To this day

I don't know, but I seemed to take on an air of independence and rarely asked for help, determined to do everything my way. That is, until it came to making my mom happy. Then I completely lost sight of myself.

It was a blustery Thursday afternoon, years later. After walking three miles from the bus stop, heavily laden backpack curving my spine into the letter "C," I entered the house to find my mom elated.

"Honey, I'm so excited," she said, grabbing the bag off my shoulders and dropping it to the floor. "I found the perfect junior prom dress for you today at the mall."

"What?" The dance was over a year away. It was the last thing on my mind.

"It's white with an empire waist and it's sleeveless." Her eyes twinkled with joy. "There are tiny blue and green flowers around the neckline and diamonds too. You're going to look like a princess!"

You've got to be kidding me, I thought. It was the middle of my sophomore year. How could my mother be thinking about the junior prom? I wasn't sure I'd even be going to the dance, let alone whether I wanted to look like a princess.

"If we leave right now, I'll have just enough time to get dinner ready."

"Mom, I have homework."

"Jackie, here's your coat." Mom threw it to me from the closet.

"I'm tired. Besides, I feel fat. Please, don't make me try anything on right now."

"I'll be waiting for you in the car."

"Mom . . . " My voice faded as she rushed out the door, the hard-driven determination in her body obvious.

Ten minutes later, we arrived at the mall. Walking several feet ahead of me, Mom marched into an obscure dress shop and grabbed the gown off the hold rack. Herding me into the dressing room, she commanded, "Quick, honey, put this on. We only have five minutes to decide."

The vision standing before me in the mirror was something straight out of a *Friday the 13th* movie. My long greasy hair looked like a rat's nest with the rodent still in it, and my brown-and-white oxford school shoes peeked out from under the elegant hemline. Sucking in my stomach so I wouldn't break the zipper, I tried to throw my shoulders back to give the image of length in my torso. To top it all off, brown eyeliner began to drip down my cheeks as I desperately tried to hold back the tears. I was not quite the vision of loveliness my mom was looking for, but she was thrilled all the same.

"You look beautiful, sweetheart. What do you think?"

Seeing the excitement in her eyes, how could I even begin to tell her that I felt like a dork? My mother was a child of the Great Depression. In her family, there had never been extra money for anything frivolous, especially a prom dress. By the time she was in her late twenties, things were still tight financially. On the day she married my father, there was no white wedding gown. Instead, she wore a brown tweed suit that later substituted for work clothes. I'd always known she wanted me to have all the things she never did. She constantly talked about how hard her life had been and that she wanted more for me, including pretty prom dresses.

Looking into her pleading face, I whispered, "Mom, it's perfect."

I vowed at an early age, with my expulsion from dance class, that I'd never do anything to displease my mother again. I spent twenty-six years bending over backward to make her proud. But the old saying "never say never" proved true in my case.

In 1978, I met the man I was to marry and took the first step toward my true independence. This time, my astrological Capricorn stubborn streak and resolve outweighed my desire to please. This goat, born on a cold December day in 1952, was on a mountaintop all by herself.

For years, I'd done what was expected, but it never felt like it brought anyone any joy, especially me. Life in the Madden household always seemed serious. It became even more so when the beginning of my mother's many health issues, laced with bouts of severe depression, appeared on the scene when I was in my early twenties. Laughter was rare and I wanted fun, so I searched for someone who would make me laugh. In Dave Haugh, I was sure I'd found it.

I knew my soon-to-be husband would provide levity. Unfortunately, my perceived impulsive and selfish decision came with a hefty price tag. Not only did my family disapprove, so did my friends. Isolation was not something I expected to experience during my engagement period. To prove them all wrong, I held my ground.

"Jackie, you can't be serious," my mother hissed, a few days after Dave asked for my hand.

"I am. Why do you have such a problem with it?"

"He's nothing like the man I expected you to pick." She paced back and forth in front of my father's red leather chair as I sat in sadness. I'd spent my entire life seeking approval, and now with the biggest event in my life, I felt like the Statue of Liberty: defiant, stoic, and alone on an island surrounded by turbulent waters.

"So, what was your vision? Some blond Adonis like that guy you liked in high school? Bart?"

Taking a moment to compose herself before she really blew, Mother lowered her voice a notch.

"Look, honey! He's like a bull in a china shop, always knocking everything over. He comes from money and you don't, and he's not Catholic," she rambled. But soon the acceleration in her voice took over, and she exploded. "Oh, for God's sake, he's even a *Republican!*"

As I was getting ready to walk down the aisle, so were several of my girlfriends. With their engagements came excitement, fanfare, and lavish bridal showers. For me, it was rarely discussed except for the occasional, "Are you sure? You can change your mind, you know."

Six months before the big day, September 15, 1979, Mom realized I was going to go through with it. There was no turning back.

"Jackie, you're getting married in just a few months," she whimpered, her voice cracking between sniffles. "We better start looking for a dress."

"Are you sure you want to do this?" I inquired, thinking perhaps I should go alone.

"Time is running out." Avoiding eye contact, she looked out the window to children playing kick the can in the street. "We need to get this done."

Shopping had become a glorious activity we shared to escape just another boring sporting event blaring from the TV on Sunday afternoons. One of the greatest gifts God gave women in the 1960s was an open mall seven days of the week. It was our time for bonding, sharing thoughts, and discovering new elements for friendship between us. But it quickly became pure hell as we searched one store after the other for my wedding dress.

Several days later, we found it at last: a simple, sleeveless empire-waist gown with white flowers encircling the neckline. I looked like a princess.

"What do you think?" I said, afraid the floodgates would open and my mom's tears would overtake the moment. But for one brief second, she looked pleased.

"You look lovely, honey." Dropping her head to find a handkerchief in her purse, she confessed, "I'm sorry this has been so hard for me. I never dreamed your wedding or the man you'd choose would be such a difficult thing for me to handle."

Watching her dissolve once again, I sat next to her on the viewing couch and wrapped her in my arms. Holding her close, I reassured her, "I know I'm doing the right thing. Please try to trust me."

From the moment I started dating at sixteen, I'd always known it would be difficult for any man I chose to be accepted by my family. Each poor soul who dared to ask me out had to first get past my brothers before he even met my parents. Unless my family was allowed to handpick a husband for me as was done in centuries long ago, it was obvious to me no one would ever be considered good enough.

While my brothers may have been rough in some areas, I always knew they adored me and wanted to protect me. In my parents' eyes, I was their delicate flower who deserved perfection. Their rose among three thorns. But nothing is ever perfect, and when it came to this most important decision, I realized that I had to do what was ultimately right for me.

For the next twenty-two years, my children's father and I built a life together. I was completely committed to the pledge I made during our wedding vows. My home was my castle, and I wanted to protect it and those I loved. Through my husband and kids, I searched for the love I felt I had missed in my youth, but it came at a hefty price.

To show my love and devotion to all, I became a gourmet caterer—not of food, but of attention to everyone's needs. I was driven to make their world a better place and to keep peace at all costs. I was compliant about any decision that needed to be made. It was calmer and much easier for everyone else to decide, even if it was on my own behalf. In other words, the girl with steel running through her veins on her wedding day had somehow turned into milk toast.

"Mom, where do you want to go for dinner on your birthday?" my daughter Lauren asked one morning in December 1992. I was about to turn forty and still wanted whatever it took to make all the members of my family pleased.

"Anywhere, sweetie. I don't care."

Stepping away from the family computer, Lauren came face-to-face with her indecisive mother. Grabbing my shoulders, she shook me firmly. "No, I want to know. It's your day! Where do you want to go?"

"Really, I don't care," I answered, afraid I'd pick someplace they didn't like.

"Fine! Then we're going to Burger King," she spat, knowing how much I hated fast food.

Assuming the role of a good girl set me on a track that would have me searching for *me* most of my life. I needed purpose and looked for it in making things wonderful for everyone else. I was fearful of anger: my husband's, my children's, my mother's, even my own. I was also frightened of rejection and the feeling of abandonment that comes with it. If I did not please my family, they just might not want anything to do with me. A healthy self-esteem eluded me once again. I never believed I could be loved for just me, and not for what I did.

But with my mother's passing, I realized that I'd wasted too many years of my life worrying about what it would take to be noticed, respected, and loved.

Despite the fact that my mom liked things a certain way, the one thing I never doubted was her deep love for me and her belief in my abilities.

As I kissed Mom good-bye for the last time on July 20, 2003, I remembered how she used to tell me, "In order to be loved, we must first love ourselves." It wouldn't be long before I discovered the love within had been right there all the time. I just needed to find the golden key, unlock the vault, and let it come out.

The Mime

With a snap of her bony wrist, Sister Mary Fidelas ripped off a piece of her lethal weapon for enforcing silence. She strategically slapped the gooey, gray duct tape across my gaping mouth, the corners firmly pressed onto my fourteen-year-old face.

"Jackie, I've had enough of your whispering," the wicked witch of the convent yelled, slamming the bolt of adhesive on my desk after finishing her job. "Maybe this will shut you up!"

Oh please God, not here too!

Once again, my desire to be heard was silenced. Would I ever find a place where I could let my words flow? Obviously, it wasn't in dance class long ago. And school seemed to have its rules too. But the truly sad thing was that no matter how hard I tried, I was even denied my voice at home—the one place everyone should feel free to talk—by overzealous, boisterous counterparts in their quest to expound about their day first. I had things to say, but it felt like nobody wanted to listen.

At home, my mother was the master of verbal communication. In other words, she did all the talking. When my older brother, David, reached critical thinking age, which for him was about four, he ran a close second. Soon, my two younger brothers chimed in the chorus, and I was left in the wings behind the curtain with no script. Oh, I had thoughts, but with the never-ending banter in our house, I couldn't get anyone to listen.

"Boys, stop fighting," Mom yelled. "Your shouting is giving me a headache."

"Mom, can I talk to you?" I called. I was standing in the doorway of our family room, waiting for the argument to turn physical.

"He started it," Tim cried.

"I don't care who started what. You're both driving me crazy!"

"Mom, I need you," I attempted again.

"Shut up, you little baby," David bellowed back. "You don't have to always be such a tattletale."

"Damn it to hell," Mom screamed. "Both of you, to your rooms!"

Stomping into the living room to decompress (although I sometimes wondered if it was more to decompose), my mother looked as if she wished she could rot away and be swept up in the tornado of our explosive home. To be blown out the door far, far away would bring peace and quiet to her frazzled nerves.

"Mom?" Again I struggled to get her attention, but from a safe distance on the other side of the door.

"Not now, Jackie." Mom stared out the window to the open field across the street. "Just give me a minute."

Without a sound, I turned and walked back to my room, shutting my door tightly. Looking at myself in the mirror, tears glossing over my ten-year-old eyes, I proceeded to tell myself about the horrible day I had at school.

"I spent the entire recess all by myself again today. No one even wanted to sit next to me at lunch." Standing there, gazing face-to-face with my ponytailed image, it was nice to think someone was listening, even if it was only me.

In those formative years of grammar school, when children gather the eggs of knowledge and put them in their Easter basket to draw upon later in life, my mother occasionally encouraged me to talk: that is, when she had the time to listen. But instead of trying to listen to what I was saying, her method of communication was the grilling technique of a presidential debate. Feeling like I was in a confrontation instead of a conversation, I became frustrated by the interrogation and I quickly shut down in silence.

I suffered from a developmental misstep along the way known as spoken clarity. I knew what was going on inside my head, but could never find the right words to express it. Weary with my lack of verbal prowess, my mom would spray me with a million questions to help me get to my point. Unfortunately, rather than helping further the cause, I closed the shutters inside my head and I went blank.

"Jackie, honey, is there anything you want to talk about? Do you have questions you need answered?"

"No, Mom. I'm fine."

Trailing me from one room to another, she'd persist. "Now, Jackie, you know you can talk to me, right?"

"Yes, Mom, I know."

"You're sure there's nothing you want to discuss?" she persisted, as her X-ray vision attempted to burn a hole through the internal iron safe where I kept all my secrets.

"No, Mom. Really there's not."

With an air of irritation, she crossed her arms over her ample bosom and gave me her famous stink-eye, as if to indicate I was lying. "There has to be *something* you need to talk about."

Of course there were things I wanted to get off my chest, but I needed to just say them and be done. There were relationship issues with friends, struggles with teachers, feelings of inadequacy with my schoolwork, and questions about religion—such as the trouble I was having understanding the mumbo jumbo taught by our pastor on his frequent visits to our classroom—the same teachings my parents had no problem accepting.

I hated getting the third degree under her intense spotlight. What would begin as conversation turned into an endless self-evaluation of *Why is it so hard for me to spit the words out? They're in my mind, but I can never say them.*

"Mom, there's nothing. Thank you!"

When I entered junior high school, I realized it was time I learned to somehow open up. Higher education meant responding in class, and whispering obviously wasn't going to work. The taste of glue across my lips was becoming even too much for me to handle. So, the burning question became where to practice this fine art.

At thirteen, I decided the best place to start was perhaps at the family dinner table.

Maybe I'll get lucky. Tonight I'm going to try to tell everyone what happened at school, I thought as I headed down the long hallway to the family meal.

With Lyndon Baines Johnson at the country's helm in 1967, the world was in a state of chaos due to the Vietnam War. New footage of the violence and insanity played before us on television every night during the dinner hour. Visions of bombs dropping and soldiers covered in blood, as they scurried with their weapons into bunkers, resembled a rerun from some old black-and-white Hollywood movie. Only this time, John Wayne wasn't in command. It was real, and all graphically illustrated on the six o'clock news.

My father was a captain in the Naval Reserves. Like almost all men at that time, he had been a soldier in World War II. Being a good and loyal American, he had his definite opinions about why we should be in the jungles of Asia. David—then a freshman at Bellarmine High School, a Jesuit institution where the mind was trained to delve deep into serious thought and emotion—had his own opinions.

"Dad, this war is stupid. We shouldn't be there," he stated in an argumentative tone, while still trying to be respectful.

My father's blood pressure was mounting and his face turned a brilliant shade of crimson. He responded in a condescending manner: "David, what do you know? It's the job of America to protect the weak."

Turning around to the television in the adjacent family room, my brother pointed to the mayhem that was being shown at that very moment. "Not when our men are getting slaughtered and no one can win. This is insane!"

For months, their discussion was replayed every evening, shortly after the sign of the cross was made and the blessing said. If I were lucky, the two of them would quickly have their say and move on to another, less volatile subject. More often than not, the argument became hostile, with neither side willing to back down.

As fists pounded the table, I could feel the invisible shrapnel spray over the table and land in my lap. Being the eternal pacifist, I hated conflict, any conflict. Each time a voice was raised in our home, I retreated inside my thick, turtle-like shell. Dinner was bad enough with Mom's lousy cooking. Why did the conversation always have to add to the evening's indigestion?

If it wasn't the hot-tempered discussion of politics, or report cards that came home unfavorable, it was the ticking time bomb one of my other two brothers would sneak to the table to disrupt this sacred family affair. In only a matter of minutes, there'd be another explosion of words, forcing me to recoil further back in my seat and zip my lips tighter. As the boys grew older, the alpha-male phenomenon took over. Soon it became a battle over who would be the dominant animal controlling the conversation.

I detested our family hour. In the quiet of my bedroom I often studied Norman Rockwell's painting on Thanksgiving and wondered if other people really ate like that. Were my family members the only ones who resembled our predecessors, the cavemen?

At the dinner table, Tim, often mistaken for my twin, sat to my left. In actuality, we couldn't have been more polar-opposite. Physically, we looked alike: freckled faces, chubby cheeks, stocky bodies, and hair the color of golden summer wheat with just a tinge of red. But Tim constantly fidgeted as if he had just sat on an anthill. It was a struggle for him to get through any meal without falling off his chair. Along with his nervous energy, incoherent sentences rambled out of his mouth as he spoke faster than he could think. He kept trying to get a line or two in before someone else spoke.

"Stop it, Tim," Mom shouted constantly. "You're going to break the chair by leaning backward. And what are you trying to say? I don't understand a word of it."

Across the cluttered table sat David, the scholar and sage who was born with a thesaurus for a brain. To the right of him, Michael.

Mature beyond his years, David was a master of the English language, always scrutinizing the meaning behind every multisyllabic word. I was mesmerized by his art of storytelling and sat in awe as he made the simplest event sound like a chapter out of an Ernest Hemingway novel. He was also an incessant tease. Because of his fast thinking, he constantly shot remarks at me rapid-fire, just to watch me squirm as I struggled to respond.

"Jackie, you know you were adopted, don't you?"

"What?"

"Mom and Dad wanted a daughter, so they found you in an orphanage."

"Stop it, Dave. That isn't true!" I glared at him.

"No, it's true. They looked all over for just the right girl who resembled the rest of us," he persisted, his face twitching to keep from bursting out in laughter. "You were left in a box on the doorstep of the home for waifs and strays. Mom and Dad rescued you." Watching my body stiffen, he added, "Sorry, but your real last name is Smith."

"Stop it, Dave. You're the only one with brown hair, so maybe you're the one adopted," I cried, not knowing what else to say to defend myself.

Michael was a beautiful child who could do no wrong. The entire family adored him. He had the face of an angel straight from a Rembrandt painting. His brilliant blue eyes, snow-white blond, curly hair, tiny nose, and deep dimples mesmerized everyone. And, just like Dave, he had a flair for flamboyant speech and teasing repartee. People were drawn to him like flies to flypaper and were enthralled with his antics.

God, this isn't fair! Why does he get all the attention? I asked in my nightly prayers. *Not only is he funny, but he's prettier than I am!*

When Dave and Michael got going with one of their vaudeville acts at dinnertime, there was no room for anyone else to climb onto the stage. The comedic dynamic duo resembled an Abbott and Costello routine, complete with slapstick gestures that knocked food onto the floor.

"Boys, calm down," Mom began. "You don't have to be so loud."

"Does anyone want to hear about my day?" I tried to cut in.

"God damn it," Dad bellowed, lowering his head further, shoveling his food into his mouth. "Can't a man ever eat in peace?"

As my mom slapped her hand on the table in an attempt to make her sons cease and desist, milk spewed across the brown Formica top and dribbled off the edge.

"Stop it!" she now screamed. Still, the pandemonium continued. I sat speechless, petting the dog that was hiding under my feet.

My parents not only sat at opposite ends of the table, they were also total opposites of each other. I often wondered how this Mutt and Jeff show ever got together, let alone got married.

My father was the epitome of the strong and silent type. Fully gray at the age of forty, Jack Madden was often mistaken for the handsome actor Spencer Tracy. Like other fathers in the 1950s and 60s, it was his role to go to work and earn money for his family. He rarely asked us questions about our day. Years later, he told me that late at night, in the private domain of their bedroom, he would grill my mother on what was happening in our lives. But not knowing that at the time, I thought he didn't care.

My mother, on the other hand, was a passionate woman who was never at a loss for discussion, statements, or questions. A child born to silent movie actors, Lassie definitely had a flair for the dramatic. Discourse seemed to be not only her way of drawing attention to herself, but also a way of releasing the pressure and tension that came with raising four children. As she let off steam, her sentences pummeled us one right after the other like a one-two punch.

"Guess who I ran into today?" Then, as if a torpedo had hit the family ship, she would shout orders. "Mike, stop kicking Dave under the table. Tim, sit still! Jackie, stop feeding the dog your dinner. I see you!" Retrieving her calm demeanor, she'd continue, "Jack, how was your day?"

Slowly my brothers' rumble would swell and, with it, so would the tone in her voice. "Tim, what is *wrong* with you? David, stop using those foul words at the table. Michael, I told you to stop!"

Listening to her was like watching a tennis match where only one dominant player controlled the game. Her lines would fly from one side of the court to the other, served with such force there was no way to return a retort before the next volley began.

What I'd hoped would be a practice field for articulation transformed into something else entirely. Instead of being a major player, I became more like the pitiful benchwarmer who sat on the sidelines watching the game but never got to play. I'd wait patiently in silence for my rowdy teammates to settle down, with my head lowered and hands in my lap.

"Does anyone want to hear about my day?" I tried to interject one night. "I heard a funny joke at lunch."

No response.

"I got a good grade on my math test."

No response.

"I'm going to run for class office."

Still no response.

"I think I'd like to jump off the Golden Gate Bridge and kill myself," I snarled, hoping that would create some attention.

"Oh, Jackie dear, did you try to say something?" Mom replied, finally. "Yes, I love that bridge too. Now who wants dessert?"

Realizing that the skill for expressing my thoughts, feelings, and dreams was quite possibly hopeless, I retreated to the sanctuary behind my bedroom door and turned to writing. My white, leather diary with lock and key, hidden under the mattress, became the absolute keeper of my precious thoughts. I poured my heart and soul out for most of my life in that gold-trimmed six-by-six-inch book.

I feel so inadequate all the time, I began, but soon hesitated and put my pen down, not knowing how to continue.

My greatest childhood fear was the idea of spending the rest of my life not being able to express myself and living only in my head.

Fallen Angel

I crawled out of the hard wooden pew where I was supposed to sit quietly that Friday night during Lent in 1957 and tiptoed to my father's side. Mystified, I wondered why my father was bowing to a picture of a half-naked man. What I didn't foresee was that this moment of confusion in this candle-lit church was something that would haunt me for years to come.

As my father slowly moved from one painting to the next, he respectfully bowed his head and recited words that made no sense, something about "Mary and the Lord is with thee." All the while, he rubbed the worn black beads of his antique rosary.

Lightly pulling on his gray woolen sweater sleeve, I whispered, "Daddy, what are you saying when you look at those pictures?"

Stopping for a moment, he turned to five-year-old me. "I'm praying to God, honey. See that man up there with the cross? That's Jesus. He died for us."

I noticed a series of paintings on the wall, each picture appearing to continue from the one before, but the story they were telling looked scary. In the first scene, a man with a beard and a golden ring hovering above his head was surrounded by a group of angry people. A crown of sharp thorns had been smashed to his forehead, blood dripping into his eyes and down his sad face.

"Why did this man have to die? Who said so?" I asked.

"Jesus is the Son of God, and his Father wanted him to die to save us from sin."

Confused, I tried to piece all this information together in the silence of my young head. God had a son whom He wanted dead because of something called sin. I was always told that fathers loved their children. How could He let this happen?

"Daddy, what's sin?" I asked, looking at the floor for fear of the answer. I knew it had to be bad and wondered if I'd ever done it.

"It's when you do something really awful that upsets God. Like when you're naughty and it makes me mad."

Thinking back to the few times my dad had yelled at me, I started to tremble with fear. Was refusing to go to bed on time or fighting with my brothers a sin? Could that make my father angry enough that he'd want me out of his life? "Daddy, didn't God love His son?"

I think Dad realized his explanation was making no sense. Since I'd yet to start my religious education in school, he began with my first lesson in Catholicism.

"Jesus is the Son of God. He's also God. God the Father sent His only Son here because He loves us so much and wants us all to go to heaven when we die. We can't get there if we have sin."

"So there are two Gods? Which one is the boss?"

"There are actually three: God the Father, God the Son, and God the Holy Ghost."

"One's a ghost?" I blurted, looking up at the vaulted ceilings to see if I could see Him flying.

My dad slid his fingers through his prematurely graying hair. He bent down, gently put his hands on my shoulders to look me straight in the eye, and said, "There is only one God. It's called the Divine Trinity, three in one. You just have to have faith in order to believe."

He then took my hand and walked me up to the altar to kneel and pray. An ornate mantel was adorned with gold candlesticks and flowers.

Pictures of flying baby angels and Jesus drifting up through a cluster of clouds were painted on the wall behind it. Peeking over my shoulder, I looked back to the long hall and noticed other devoted followers, crossing their foreheads with their fingertips and bending down on one knee. It seemed they too had this thing call faith, but how? The story my dad was telling sounded like some scary fairy tale of kings and talking animals written by the Brothers Grimm. How was I expected to believe in something that didn't feel real?

That evening while crawling into bed, I thought about how peaceful my dad looked in that church. At home, he was always working around the house, annoyed when we got in his way. He rarely laughed or even talked, but in that palace made only for God, he seemed to find serenity, even joy. I was determined to be just like him, but I was having a difficult time with the three-in-one description. Could it be like the Certs candy mints I'd steal from my mom's purse? The slogan said it was "Two, two, two mints in one." Maybe because God was more important he needed extra help to get his job done.

In our little bedroom community of San Carlos, it felt like the entire town was Catholic. My paternal grandmother, with her thick Irish brogue, loved to remind me it was the only true religion.

Mumbling her daily prayers as she rocked away, staring out the living room window to my mother's rose garden, she wore her rosary beads thin. "Jackie, you need to learn to be a good Catholic. We're the special, chosen people God loves the most."

"But what about all the other children who don't go to our church?" I asked, thinking of the few kids I knew from other schools. "God must love them too."

"Those are pagan babies and have black souls," Grandma answered with noticeable disgust, continuing to rock to the steady beat of her recited Hail Marys. "They may not get into heaven."

Horrified, I looked into the face of this stout Irish matriarch and wondered why God didn't love all little children. Afraid that I might end up in hell with all those with dirty souls, I vowed to live a clean and pure life. Sin was not something I'd ever commit. I was already the good child at home. It soon became my mission to be the perfect little girl, not only in the eyes of my parents, but in God's eyes too. But first, I needed to learn the rules. I had to find that thing called faith.

One Sunday morning after Mass, at the age of six, I approached my father as he sat in his leather chair hidden behind the morning newspaper. I approached, determined to set my sail on the right course. "Dad, what are some of the different sins?"

"Well, if you rob, cheat, or kill someone, that's a sin. If you laugh or talk in church, or have impure thoughts, that's one too," he replied absently. He peeked over the top of his Sporting Green. "Jackie, just know that if it's not good behavior, it's a sin, so don't do it."

Walking away, I thought: *if a sin is a sin no matter what it is, and I'm going to be equally punished, then I might as well make it a big one if I ever decide to make God mad.* Stealing money from my dad's wallet would be far more beneficial than giggling in church. At least for a short time, I'd have fun buying some toys with my newfound income before I went to hell.

I was beginning to understand the church's demands for living a life of grace, but it was all the other trappings that went with it I found to be too much for one little girl to handle.

I found rising early each Sunday morning to be at Mass by 8:00 painfully tedious. Staying home in my pajamas and playing with my dolls was far more fun than being shoved into a frilly dress and having every hair on my head plastered into place. However, I did appreciate that it was the day of the week that belonged to those three guys (in one) who lived somewhere called heaven. If I wanted good things to happen to me, then I better show up.

As I got down on my knees each night before bedtime, my parents reminded me that God could hear my prayers and would answer them. I was in the first grade, and there was a whole Christmas list I needed to pray for. Barbie longed for a car, as well as several new outfits, if she were to remain the best-dressed toy in my room. So, dutifully off to church I went, with the long list tucked deep within my coat pocket as a reminder.

But I had a difficult time accepting all the other parts of my religion. The men of God who ran things at the Vatican loved to impose suffocating rules that they claimed were to aid our rich, moral living. While my mother was definitely strict, even she didn't have as many restrictions as the church seemed to have. Life can be hard enough when you're a child, what with homework, trying to be noticed and appreciated by your family, plus constantly cleaning your room. Why did Catholicism have to make it worse?

There was fasting before receiving Communion, which always gave me a headache as well as a growling stomach. No meat on Fridays left me with heartburn due to my mom's inability to cook frozen breaded fish sticks without burning them. Giving up something I loved for Lent (which usually meant candy) made me crave sugar the way a junkie needs a fix. Even my attire was regulated. Topping off the Sunday best with a wire-brimmed hat made my head itch as if a swarm of lice had made a new home underneath.

But the worst had to be the guilt. In Catholicism, if you didn't feel bad about *something*, you were doing something wrong. There was guilt for having nice clothes, guilt for Santa Claus being generous on Christmas. Hell, there was even guilt for having food on the table.

"Jackie, it's a sin to leave food on your plate. You should be grateful you have dinner," Mom seemed to say every evening as I picked at my food, shoving the morsels from one side of the plate to the other. "There are children starving in China."

Looking at the typical evening meal of overcooked vegetables and mystery meat hidden in a brown gooey sauce, I thought: *I'd be happy to mail it to them.*

But to pour hot tar over the already burning pavement under my toes, the nuns at my grammar school made me want to throw up my hands and cry, "Uncle!"

During those early school years at St. Charles, children were beaten over the head daily with how our lives were supposed to run. Every action we made had a sin attached to it, even if you were only thinking it. Just one slip-up, and off to hell you were bound.

In a sea of green-and-blue plaid uniforms and highly shined shoes, children were expected to behave according to the plan. There was no room for individuality. Crossing the line in appearance, thought, word, or deed was cause for severe punishment.

On Monday mornings, during the religious portion of our studies, Sister Mary Peter would first ask the frightening question, "Who actually went to Mass Sunday?" Inevitably, one student would slip and tell the truth: that they had stayed home and watched cartoons. After a tongue-lashing on the evils of laziness on the Sabbath, we were led straight to her favorite subject, sin.

"All right, children," she shouted. "Let's review. What is sin?"

"Sin is anything that goes against God and His teachings," we all resounded mechanically.

"How many forms of sin are there?"

"There are two, mortal and venial," I chimed with the other forty-nine children. Then I remembered the original sin that Adam and Eve committed. They were our first dysfunctional parents, who'd screwed up big time. Because of their actions, children came into this world already damaged and needing to be bathed immediately in baptism.

"Excuse me, Sister," I called out, my hand reaching for the ceiling. "I don't understand how eating an apple is such a bad thing."

"Because God told them not to eat the forbidden fruit."

"Does that mean I shouldn't eat the apple my mom put in my lunch bag?"

Sister Mary Peter tapped her hand with the long pointer she often used on children who asked stupid questions. "Did God tell you not to eat it?"

Knowing I was about to get whacked, I didn't go any further.

I couldn't help but wonder if anyone ever really heard God. I knew He never talked to me. I was constantly trying, but He wasn't answering. I even sank so low as to barter with Him to get his attention.

God, if you make Janie my friend, I promise I'll be a good girl.

God, if I get a bike for Christmas, I promise I'll be a good girl forever.

God, if you make me beautiful, I will never ask for another thing in my life.

While I couldn't completely wrap myself around Sister Mary Peter's nonsensical teachings, I knew I had a spiritual side. I instinctively believed there had to be a power greater than myself simply by watching all the beauty in the world. Every day I searched to find it. When I heard the coo of a mourning dove or saw a bud opening for the first time, I knew that this person called God must be close by.

"Mom, I'm sure I saw Him today," I shouted, running through the front door after school one day, going straight for a glass of milk and a cookie. I was in the second grade, and my First Holy Communion was in a couple of months. I looked for Him everywhere.

"Who?"

"God!"

"You did? Where was He?" Mom asked, trying not to laugh.

"He was in the sky," I began, out of breath with excitement. "Thick clouds were slowly going away, and a beautiful ray of light beamed straight down onto the schoolyard. Then there was a giant rainbow."

"It sounds beautiful."

"It was the most amazing sight I've ever seen. That had to be God, right?"

Kissing my cheek, Mom wrapped her arms around me, and said, "Yes, sweetie. God is everywhere."

But as I grew older, I found myself getting disillusioned, even angry, at the church. My higher education was preparing me for critical thinking, but my religious training was asking me to accept without question. In high school, I began to tear apart all the stories I was taught in my youth.

On a warm fall afternoon in the ninth grade, I stormed into the house to confront my mother with my latest discovery of what I perceived to be just another lie. At Mercy High School, religious instruction wasn't the only piece to the curriculum. There was sex education too.

"Mom, let's talk about the Immaculate Conception."

"Yes, honey. What about it?"

"So, Mary did it with the Holy Spirit?"

Mom looked up from folding the laundry. "Excuse me?"

"Well, all these years I've been told she was a virgin. She had to get that sperm in her somehow. They say it was the Holy Ghost."

"That's the teaching of the church," Mom stammered. "You need faith to believe."

"Come on, that makes no sense. I'm not stupid," I yelled, throwing my hands up in the air. "I know how babies are born."

The worst incrimination imposed by the church was over my budding sexuality. I couldn't understand why God gave us erratic hormones and

animal urges, but we weren't allowed to explore them. It seemed the cruelest of all tortures.

"You know, Jackie, it's a sin to have sex before marriage," my mom warned from the moment I became a woman at fourteen. "You have to save yourself for your husband."

"Yeah, Mom. I know."

"It's also a sin to French kiss a boy."

Looking up from my schoolwork, I thought back to the recent dance where Rick and I had swapped spit on the dance floor. "Why is that a sin?" I asked, trying to avoid eye contact.

"Because one minute you're kissing and the next he has his hand up your skirt," she answered in an agitated voice. "That's how girls get pregnant."

"Oh, please." I sighed and rolled my eyes.

"Just don't let anyone touch you inappropriately. In fact, don't let anyone touch you at all!"

Finally, in college I gave up. I stopped trying to be like my parents. Once I got the opportunity to make my own decisions, I turned my back on my upbringing. I stopped praying, I stopped believing, and most of all, I stopped talking to God. He didn't seem to listen anyway.

It would be years later before I shamefully tiptoed back into a house of worship. I was a single working girl in San Francisco, and my hedonistic lifestyle felt shallow. Something was missing amidst the late nights out, drinking, partying, and dancing in nightclubs. My life was empty, and I knew it was more than the lack of a boyfriend. My soul seemed to be crying out for fulfillment. So, back to my roots I went, only this time it would be on my terms.

Okay, God. I'm here, I prayed, kneeling in the poorly lit sanctuary of St. Mary's Cathedral where my parents had been married. *But this time I'm doing it my way. I refuse to feel guilty any longer.*

I planned to follow the teachings of Christ and Christ alone. I would now decide what was morally right for me, even if the church vehemently disapproved.

Years later, I hoped my children could get something out of religion even if I didn't. Unsure how to go about giving them the opportunity, I found myself repeating my past as each baby was born. I hoped that Catholic instruction and approach had changed and that faith could be explained better and communicated more fully.

My mother and I were sitting at my kitchen table, having coffee. I confessed: "I can't believe I'm sending Michelle to a Catholic grammar school. I hated St. Charles, and vowed I'd never do that to one of my own."

"Honey, you're doing the right thing," she said. "The real world can be a big and scary place, and you can't be with your children every second of every day. They need something to hang onto that gives them comfort when they're young." Looking into her cup, she confessed, "My faith hasn't been that easy. You haven't been alone in your struggles."

Shocked, I stared at my mother. Like my father, she was a rule follower. She'd always appeared to be happy in the process of devoting her life to doing God's work as she attended to the needs of others, putting her own needs on the back burner.

"Really? But you never complained about it like I do."

"That's just what our generation did. We were raised to accept and not question."

I've often wondered if children bear the sins of their parents. In my case, there were no sins to be passed on to the Madden kids. God couldn't have placed two more loving and ethical human beings on the face of this earth. My mother and father lived their lives by the Bible and obeyed all the rules. Unfortunately, my children's mother was not quite so perfect.

In my quest to discover my place in the spiritual world, I made several horrible mistakes and allowed myself to be sucked up into situations that went against God's plan or what was considered to be socially acceptable. One particular decision would torture me for the rest of my life.

I was engaged, and the wedding was four months away. The dress was ordered, the invitations were carefully being addressed, and the nonrefundable down payment for the reception at the Stanford Faculty Club had been submitted. My mother had finally accepted that I was going to go through with the plan and actually began to show signs of excitement.

Dave had moved to San Diego a month after he proposed to take a job he hoped would cement our financial future. We saw each other only on weekends.

Early one Monday morning in March 1979, a little pink cross magically appeared on the drugstore vial after I realized my cycle was a month behind schedule. I panicked. Good girls didn't get pregnant before they got married. This news would not only humiliate my mother, but devastate her as well. To her, I'd always been her pure and shining star. Her rose, forever in full bloom. Staring at my horrified reflection in the bathroom mirror, I'd never felt so alone.

"Dave, I'm pregnant," I cried hysterically into the phone.

"What? Weren't you using protection?"

Once again I felt like I had failed, and it was all my fault. All I could say was: "Yes. But obviously it didn't work."

The silence on the other end of the phone was deafening. Then, in a barely audible voice, Dave said: "Jackie, I'll support whatever you want to do, but I'd rather we didn't have a baby now."

For weeks I sobbed, tossed, and turned. I had no one to talk to and didn't know where to go for help. In 1979, personal predicaments of this nature were not discussed among friends. Private matters remained just that, private. I wanted to return to the days when I was a little girl and could hide under my bed to wait for the bad things to go away.

I tried to tell my mother, but all she talked about was how perfect and beautiful my wedding was going to be. Pastel pink dresses on the bridesmaids, white tuxes on the groomsmen, the little rosebuds I'd wear in my hair. This would be the wedding my mother never had, and she was determined to make everything flawless. The image of a bulging tummy as I walked down the aisle was not in the plans. Later, my parents would have to deal with the questions from the town gossipmongers.

"Did you hear Jackie Madden delivered a baby four months premature?" I could just hear the tongues wagging. "Funny thing is, it weighed eight pounds. Doesn't sound premature to me."

Image and the good family name were essential for my mom. It was as important as the air she breathed. "Jackie, your reputation is everything in life," she liked to remind me constantly. "If you don't have that, you have nothing." In my devastated heart, I was sure this would kill her.

As I neared the end of the first trimester, I started to spot. Throughout the day, the telltale sign that something was wrong was evident each time I used the restroom. *Oh my God! Am I having a miscarriage?* I wondered, as the cramping became severe.

But the following day all was back to normal. The amusement park roller coaster ride I was on had me jerked in so many directions that my neck was suffering from whiplash. The sleepless nights left me looking as if I was at death's door, dark circles under my eyes and pale in complexion, and every part of my body ached from tension and fear.

I wanted to keep the baby. Being a mother was all I'd ever dreamed about. But I was terrified by what the news might do to my mother. Her health was beginning to deteriorate and she was in constant pain. To top it off, my parents were dealing with drugs, alcohol, and anger management issues with Michael, then eighteen. He was a constant worry. I couldn't let this good girl be added to the list of my parents' disappointments.

I made the decision to terminate, a decision I will regret until the day I die. I made a call to Planned Parenthood. With a mere four hundred dollars, a child was lost forever.

For the next six years, I lived in my own private hell, as I lay in bed at night wondering who that little person might have been. I worried that I was doomed for damnation at the end of my days. The church has strict rules against abortion. Just when I felt as if I was finding my faith, I feared I was about to be excommunicated. I couldn't go on living in the hell I'd created for myself. I needed forgiveness.

I was about to give birth to my third child, Lauren, when I went to visit the priest who'd married Dave and me. He was a close friend of my parents.

"Bless me, Father, for I have sinned." Crying hysterically, I told him everything.

He put his arms around me and held me tight.

"Will I still be able to raise my children as Catholics?" I trembled.

His gentle, soothing manner calmed my sobs. He said, "God forgave you long ago when he blessed you with all these children. It's time you forgive yourself and put this behind you."

Wiping the tears from my eyes, I realized he was right. Not only had God given me two healthy, wonderful little girls, a third was on its way. I'd been given a second chance to be the mother I always wanted to be. God wasn't a vengeful deity, but truly loving and forgiving.

My children know about my mistakes. We've talked at great lengths about the choices life puts in front of us, and where to turn when faced with difficult decisions. I felt intensely alone during those days. Now that I'm older, I realize my mother would have survived the news. It definitely would have taken its toll, but she was stronger than I sometimes gave her credit for when it came to what the neighbors thought. I can only pray my children will never be afraid to come to me.

When my four children make their mistakes, it will not be my place to judge them, and I'll have to put my own ego aside. It will be my duty and responsibility to help them. If they're faced with something that rips their souls apart, as this decision did mine, I know God will be right at my side showing me the way to help. Life has a way of making everything all right for those who have faith.

For years I desperately wanted to have what my parents had, a life of unwavering faith. I marveled at the depth of their connection with the Lord. I often wondered why I couldn't be like them.

In the end, I came to realize it didn't matter whether we believed the same things, but that we were faithful to our beliefs and our own truths. My father honored his, my mother hers, and I mine. In the end, the Lord loves us all.

What truly matters while we are here on earth is our conviction of the heart and the life we lead. Do we care about others? Do we give of ourselves and share the gifts we have? Are we kind, considerate, loving, and loyal?

Some may think of me as a wayward Catholic because I follow my heart and not what I'm told to follow, but I do believe there'll be a place for me in heaven one day. It will be right next to both my parents and my very first child on that day when I'm called home.

Mother Incarnate

On July 22, 1981, the first of my four treasured children, Michelle, was born. With her came my reincarnation in the guise of Demeter, the Greek goddess of the harvest and original Mother Earth, queen of domestic perfection. I'd spent my whole life searching for that one thing that I would excel at, be proficient in, and act out flawlessly. At twenty-eight, I knew I'd found it: motherhood.

"I'm coming, honey. Mommy's here to take care of you," I called as I heard my baby's cries. Flying from a dead sleep to her newly decorated nursery room, I prepared myself to go into turbo mode. It was her first night home from Stanford Hospital, and I was beyond excited to prove to all concerned (especially myself) that I was indispensable.

Unfortunately, as I lifted my baby from her bed, I was punched in the stomach with a horrible realization, and an unwanted moment of truth.

Stumbling through the dark, I was about to change the first messy diaper alone. After spending the entire day with me, my mother was now nowhere to be found. It was up to me, and me alone, to clean up the gooey mess that had erupted from this magnificent specimen of babyhood.

"Yuck! What is that stuff? It looks like cottage cheese with a tan," I said out loud, as if someone would answer and say everything was just as it should be. "Is that normal?"

Hearing my child wail, I mentally turned my queasy stomach onto silent and went into action. "Okay, honey. Mommy is here to get you out of that dirty diaper."

With chubby legs kicking wildly, Michelle pursed her lips for another feeding.

"Now just relax," I whispered, quickly becoming equally agitated. "Michelle, stop wiggling."

Rolling back and forth on the changing table, she flailed her little arms as she tried to grab hold of her maternal feeding machine.

"No, you have to stay on your back for me to do this." Now I was panicking. "Stop, Michelle! Hold still. You're making me nervous." *Oh, God, please help me!* I thought. With my left elbow draped gently across her chest to lock her in place, my other hand manipulated the cotton diaper under her derriere.

Clueless, I called in the reserves. "Dave, wake up and help me. Which way does this go?"

From off in the distance, I heard a faded voice as Dave buried his head deeper into his foxhole. "How in the hell am I supposed to know?" he grunted, now completely under the covers of our bed.

"I need help! How do I get this thing on?"

"Didn't they teach you what to do in the hospital?" he snarled.

Sweat beaded at my brow. Under my arms, water ran like the Truckee River just after the snow began to melt from the Sierras.

"Dave?"

"Jackie, leave me alone. I need some sleep," Dave yelled, smashing the pillows over his head. "Someone around here has to go to work in the morning."

Oh yeah! Like I get to lie around all day.

In that moment, the cute safety pin, with the head of a yellow ducky covering the clasp, morphed into the image of a Chinese Pa Kua Dao: a forty-one-inch chrome-plated steel blade big enough to slice an elephant in half.

In this surreal instant, I felt like I was being transformed into a vicious warrior from a Chinese revolution, out to slaughter all baby girls. Holding Michelle's tiny legs up in the air, I prayed: *Please, God, where are you when I need you? I'm afraid I'm about to stab my own child.*

I was totally unprepared for this part of parenting. I began to fall apart. In that pastel pink and green nursery, with rows and rows of new stuffed animals looking on and only the soft glow of a night-light illuminating the changing table, I felt alone.

"What are you looking at?" I whispered angrily to the life-size Raggedy Ann smirking from the corner of the room. "What possessed me to think you were cute and worth adding to this menagerie?"

After the third attempt, I was sure I had everything securely pinned together. But as I lifted Michelle to my chest, the diaper fell from her body and landed on the floor.

The next try was even worse. Not only did the fluffy fabric fall, but another eruption blasted, and she exploded like Mount St. Helens down the front of my nightgown. Numerous unsuccessful tries later, exasperation and a bucket of tears surged to the surface.

I shouted at my sleeping husband: "Dave, get up and grab a paper diaper from the bag! They're sitting by the door."

With a disgusted moan, Dave crawled out of bed to retrieve the hospital-issued diapers. As he threw the easy, breezy disposable into the room, a feeling of defeat surged through my core. I'd sworn I'd never sink to the paper diaper cop-out. My baby's world was supposed to be environmentally pure. Yet with barely a flip to my nervous fingers, all my planning and research were for naught. The adhesive tabs were in place and the tears subsided. At least, Michelle's tears did.

With a baby blanket wrapped around my chest to keep the remains of the atomic detonation from soiling my daughter, Michelle was back in my arms, ready for her feeding.

"There you go, honey. All safe and sound," I cooed in her ear, as tears pooled in my eyes. *Oh dear Lord. I don't think I'm cut out for this. I want my mom.*

Rocking together slowly, we swayed to the melodic tick of the cuckoo clock down the hall. As Michelle drifted back to sleep, my thoughts of peace and serenity transformed into scenarios of all the possible "mommy failures" I might face in the future. *If I can't close a stupid diaper pin, how am I going to handle the really big issues that will come?*

In that moment, I realized perfection would not be a word used to describe my parenting skills. Considering how difficult it was to master one child, the future three we were planning would be impossible.

Instead of pretending to be little Miss Suzy Homemaker, like a lioness protecting her cubs, I would become a military helicopter. Hovering overhead, I positioned myself perfectly, ready to swoop down at a moment's notice to whisk my charges away from any possible harm.

It would be five years before I let anyone put my children to bed without me. I had no use for babysitters, those strange creatures that come in and take charge while you're out supposedly having a good time. But as my three young girls were consuming my every waking moment, I came to realize my husband needed attention too.

One Friday evening, Dave walked into the house and announced: "Jackie, enough is enough! We can't stay home every night. We need to go out once in a while."

He bent over to look for a beer in the refrigerator. "Look, I was driving down the street today and I saw a group of teenagers standing on the corner. I asked if any of them babysat. I got a few phone numbers."

I was horrified that he'd ask just anyone to babysit our kids. Especially someone on a street corner! I asked in my best pissy fashion, "So, not only are you asking me to miss one night of our girls' lives, but you want to leave them in the hands of some kid hanging out on a street corner?" My hands firmly planted on my hips, sparks flying with each breath, I prepared myself for a showdown of wills. "As far as you know, that may be how she makes all her money, holding up the lamppost, soliciting customers. And I'm not talking babysitting."

Dave just looked at me. Studying the face of the man I'd promised to love, honor, and cherish, I realized "pay attention to" needed to be included in the list of matrimonial vows. Unfortunately, that meant I'd have to spread myself even thinner if our marriage was to survive the pandemonium of child-rearing.

"Okay," I relented. "But I want to interview them."

"What's to interview? They're only thirteen years old. Just pick one," he snorted. "I can't stay home another night."

Giving into a night out was difficult, but being the dutiful, loyal, and selfless "little" woman, I made the phone call to one of the girls on Dave's list.

The following evening, a child from the underworld with black fingernail polish, fishnet stockings, and hair strangely resembling a rat's nest on the side of her head appeared on my doorstep.

"Hi, Mrs. Haugh. I'm Linda, your new babysitter."

Stunned, it took me a moment to pull myself together, though I felt I was disintegrating. "Hi, Linda. Interesting outfit. Does your mother let you buy your own clothes?" I wanted to know what kind of woman would allow her child out of the house looking like a beaten-up rock star.

In 1986, all the teenyboppers in town were turning into clones of Madonna, the latest musical sensation, who sang love ballads extolling the virtues of raw sex. Linda's clothes were an eclectic mishmash of stripes, polka dots, cheap lace, rhinestones, and netting. Around her neck were several beaded chains and an enormous crucifix that swayed back and forth, looking more like a weapon than a religious symbol. Eyeing the monstrous size of this thing, I wondered if she used it on kids when they didn't do what she asked.

Fear paralyzed me as I left my kids with this enigma, but off I went with my husband for dinner and a movie. We hadn't gone out alone since I'd been pregnant with Michelle.

"And what will the lady have tonight?" the waiter asked politely a third time, as I stared at the couple next to us. Just to my right was a happy mother and father close to our age, with their baby in the restaurant's highchair.

"Dave, why couldn't we bring the kids? They know how to behave."

"Stop it, Jackie, and order. We'll be late for the movie."

"I don't know what I want." All I'd eaten in months was hot dogs and macaroni and cheese.

As the waiter impatiently tapped his pen on his pad of paper, Dave nudged me under the table to get on with it.

"I guess I'll just have a salad. I'm not very hungry, but bring on the wine."

After the movie, some God-awful horror film with the neighborhood psychopath kidnapping babies from their beds while the parents were having a date night, I couldn't get home fast enough.

"Can you speed it up a little?"

"Jackie, relax. I'm not going to get a ticket just so you can get home five minutes sooner," Dave hissed. "I'm sure everything is fine. Linda would have called if it wasn't."

Watching the speedometer needle hit just below the speed limit, I wondered if Dave was doing this just to torture me. He never had a problem zipping home to watch a Stanford basketball game, or any other sporting event on TV.

The moment we pulled into the driveway, I jumped out of the car as if I were trying to escape a date gone bad and I was about to be faced with the possibility of kissing the creep good night. "I'm coming, kids. Mommy's home!"

Bolting through the front door, I was shocked to find that everything was quiet, clean, and in order.

"What do you mean, they didn't ask for me? No one cried when I wasn't there to kiss them good night?"

"No, Mrs. Haugh, everything went great. You have fun kids," Linda said. "We made a fort under the dining room table, ate popcorn, and watched movies." Then, adding more insult to my bruised ego, she added, "They had a healthy salad for dinner."

"A *salad?* They never eat salads or vegetables."

"Maybe you don't put enough salad dressing on them."

Whether it brought me comfort or not, I had to accept the fact that my children would survive quite nicely without me on an occasional basis.

Their father, however, had quickly become my fourth child, and did not seem to be managing as well as the toddlers. He needed a lot of consideration. Instinctively, I knew that my marriage was just as important to safeguard, and that I'd better pay attention if we were to last "until death do us part."

But leaving the kids in the hands of baby watchers was one thing. How to cope when they were physically separated from me due to circumstances beyond my control nearly brought me to ruin.

Children bring great joys, but they also come with nasty germs. Most of my kids' illnesses were run-of-the mill: flu, cold, croup, headache, and sore throat. Occasionally a more serious condition presented itself, and I had to rally all my strength to be the shining and steadfast beacon of light in the stormy port.

At ten days old, Timmy, my fourth and final child, developed a fever. I took him into the doctor's office to be checked out. I was told, "Jackie, you need to get this baby to the hospital immediately. Babies this age don't get fevers unless there is something terribly wrong." I bundled up my son and raced off to El Camino Hospital's emergency room, where he was ripped out of my arms for a battery of invasive and painful tests.

"We're not sure what's wrong with Timmy," the ER doctor said, after the examination. "He could have spinal meningitis or a bacterial blood disease."

"What do you mean you don't know what is wrong with him? He's so little. He has to be okay." Taking a breath, I mumbled, "He's my only son!"

"We will first do a spinal tap and go from there."

From behind the swinging doors, I heard my baby scream. I imagined his tiny body being stuck with five-inch long needles, and in response, the milk in my breast flooded down my body.

Later, seeing my precious son wearing only a diaper in the cold, sterile environment of the intensive care unit broke my heart. There were tubes sprouting from his tiny head and arms. I felt totally helpless for the first time in my life. I was lost as my emotions spun out of control. There was nothing I could do but stand by Timmy's crib and gently stroke his burning forehead. It would be several hours before I could hold him in my arms again.

"He looks cold. Can we put a blanket on him?" I asked, my voice quivering.

"He really isn't cold, Mrs. Haugh," his nurse replied softly, so as not to wake him. "His fever is high, and that alone is keeping him warm. But we can put a little sheet over him if that will make you feel better."

"Please. I can't stand seeing him not cuddled up in something."

My only recourse was faith, that thing my parents clung to and I found hard to find. I bartered, pleaded, begged, and prayed that God would guide the doctors with the course of action necessary to heal my son.

During those seemingly endless seven days, my life resembled a white yo-yo with a rainbow stripe down the middle. When the yo-yo came to a stop, you could see all the bright colors, but that didn't last long. Before long, it was spinning with such velocity that all the colors blurred into one.

"Jackie, slow down," Dave would yell, looking up from the TV, as I dashed out the door each night.

I had to keep my home life running smoothly as well as care for my sick child. Raising four children under the age of six meant a lot of planning. It took skill, patience, and precision to keep the schedule on track. I sped back and forth from the hospital to the house every couple of hours, to make sure the girls were eating, bathed, and in bed on time.

"Michelle, is your homework done?" I would begin, before seeing to the other two. "Jenni, Lauren, quick, get into the tub. I need to wash your hair."

"Kids, put your dishes in the sink," I'd say, grabbing my purse to leave for the fifth time that day. "Don't worry, Dave, I'll do them later when I get back. Timmy needs to be fed."

"Jackie, this is ridiculous," Dave would argue, as his whirling tornado of a wife spun in a vortex of uncontrollable energy. "Timmy is in good hands. They can take care of him when you aren't there."

"No, they can't!" I was appalled that Tim's own father didn't understand. "They can't love him the way I do. I need to be there."

"I was with him this afternoon and plan to go see him after the game is over." My husband's eyes were firmly locked on the Giants game. "Why don't you relax?"

"No, I don't want him to wait that long. Please leave a light on."

The only quiet moments during those horrific days came at Timmy's last feeding, when the hospital buzz settled down and all the sick children on the ward were fast asleep. With the usually blinding fluorescent lights dimmed, the soft rhythmic hum of the heart monitor floated in the air. The pediatric wing can be very peaceful at one o'clock in the morning.

Scooping up my tiny child in my shaking arms, careful not to dislodge any of the medical equipment, I held him close to my heart and rocked back and forth, hanging onto every second as if it might be my last.

Nine long days later, the verdict on Timmy's condition arrived. The doctor on call announced he would be just fine and could go home in a couple of hours. "We performed every possible test on your son and everything came out negative. We now believe he had an earache."

"*What?* He only had an earache?" I was astounded. "Why was that so hard to detect?"

"Babies usually don't get fevers until they're about three months old, and earaches are unheard of until four months. He is way ahead of the health schedule."

Great! That's all I need, a child who wants to push the envelope with his well-being.

I was ecstatic that my baby was fine, elated that I was about to bring him home, and thrilled at the thought I'd finally get some sleep. I wrapped my son up in his cozy blue velour blanket, nuzzled his delicate, soft throat, and whispered, "I'm going to have to keep my eye on you. I'm not letting you out of my sight."

For the sake of my children, I may have made some decisions that were not good for my marriage. I felt God had gifted us with these kids, and it was my job to see to it that they ended up the way He intended: strong, moral, productive members of society, and all in one piece.

I also knew Dave required his own playtime and craved the attention that a social setting provided. More and more often, outlets with his male companions became crucial as he found ways to leave the compound on weekends and evenings. But I had needs too.

I gave my husband permission to do whatever he wanted. I hoped he would see that it was vital for me to be successful with the job I loved the most: raising our four children. While we spent countless hours apart fulfilling our passions, I prayed that their father would understand, support me, and, hopefully, want the same thing: what was right for the kids.

Dr. Jekyll and Mrs. Hyde

One lazy Monday afternoon in 1999, my friend and I were sitting on a park bench watching Timmy play with his toddler buddies. I confided to her that I seriously thought I was going crazy. As I aggressively rubbed the roots of my short blonde hair, my frustration exploded. "I feel like my hair follicles are on fire. My migraines are out of control, and I hate everything!"

"No, you don't, Jackie. You love Dave and the kids."

"Not right now. I wish they'd all take a long trip around the world and leave me alone."

At thirty-eight-years old, I was the mother of four high-spirited hummingbirds under the age of eight, constantly flitting from one mess to another. While my youngest was only two, in my mind, I was still youthful, vibrant, and unwrinkled. I could still run faster than any of my kids to get to the bathroom first. But suddenly my demeanor was changing.

In an instant, I could go from Little Miss Sweetness and Light to a monster. One moment I was the reliable, calm, and stable mom my family could count on. The next, I was a striptease artist tearing off extra clothing that made me pour sweat.

"Mom, what are you doing?" Michelle shrieked as I threw my blouse on the floor. My nine-year-old daughter was not accustomed to witnessing her mother parade around the house in only her bra and jeans. "It's freezing in here. Can we turn on the heater?"

"Heat? Did you say heat?" I cried, wiping the sweat from my moist brow. "I'm boiling!"

"But, Mom, it's raining outside and you have all the windows open."

As she forced the sliding glass door of my bedroom shut, I looked at my perplexed daughter. "Don't do that! Here, put on my sweatshirt and stop complaining. I'm so hot I think I'm about to pass out."

Everything annoyed me in that gloomy period: fingerprints on the hallway walls, a shoe left in the middle of the room, the dog barking at strangers, my husband lying on the couch. In the heat of one of those moments, I'd go from one room to the next on a rampage.

Storming into the family room, I prepared myself for battle. "Dave, what kind of example are you setting for the kids? Get your feet off the furniture."

"Jackie, that's what couches are for," Dave replied calmly, fearful he might set off another explosion. "I'm tired and want to watch the baseball game."

"And that's another thing. All you do is lie around watching one goddamn game after another. I'm sick of it!" I stomped out the door, to avoid him getting the last word in.

Heading to the only peaceful room in the house, my bathroom, I began to choke up with the unfairness of it all. Dave worked hard at his job when our children were young. Because he was a commercial real estate broker, his income was solely commission. With four small children, he busted his hump trying to provide and plan for our financial future. He deserved to relax once in a while. He also deserved to put his feet on the furniture.

After a good, long sob, I returned to the family room to apologize. "I'm sorry. I don't know what's wrong with me."

"I think you need to go see a doctor. You haven't been yourself for a long time now," Dave said sympathetically, looking up from the Giants' ninth inning. Then he added tersely, "Whatever it is, fix it. You're driving us all crazy!"

"Yeah, Mommy," a little voice came from the other room.

My seven-year-old, Jenni—always the gentle soul in the family—appeared in the doorway afraid to enter the room. With her moon-shaped freckled face, hazel eyes, and innocent demeanor, she looked me straight in the eye, "Why are you so mad all the time?"

"I'm sorry, sweetie. I'll talk to the doctor tomorrow."

The next morning, I made the call and got the earliest possible appointment. I was sure something was seriously wrong. Was it a tumor? Was I psychotic or bipolar? Was I dying?

Two days later, sitting on the examining table, I was hopeful for some help, but fearful that I was headed for the loony bin.

"Won't anyone listen to me?" I cried to my gynecologist, as I sat on the examining table for my annual "poke and prod." Vehemently shaking my head, my hands covering my eyes to hold back the tears, I blurted, "I feel like I'm losing my mind."

"Jackie, there is nothing wrong with you. Everything is fine. I think you're probably just overloaded with all those kids," my doctor told me lightly. "Maybe you need a glass or two of wine in the evening."

"Okay, that's easy to do. But what do I do during the day?"

"Take a nap."

I stared at this distinguished man who'd brought my babies into the world. I wondered if he was the one who'd now lost his mind. "Yeah, right! Take a nap. That's a good one."

"I really think it's all in your head," the doctor suggested in his genteel bedside manner. "Perhaps you need a new attitude."

I need more than that, I thought, as I slowly got dressed. *I need a miracle.*

Leaving the office, feeling dejected, I made up my mind that from now on, only positive thoughts and words would flow from my out-of-whack body.

I drove home carefully, repeating over and over, "Stay calm, stay calm."

But somehow our house had transformed into a junkyard while I was away. Everywhere I looked, small colorful plastic Legos were strewn.

"Goddamn it! Who made this mess?" I screamed at the top of my lungs.

A little voice came from behind the overstuffed plaid chair in the corner. "I'm sorry, Mommy. I did it." My precious baby boy, fearing for his life, clutched his blanket in anticipation of my wrath.

What is wrong with me? I wondered. *How could I ever get mad at these kids, especially Timmy? This is not who I am.* "Honey, I'm sorry for yelling. Will you help me clean this up?"

Timmy toddled slowly out to me and wrapped his little arms around my knees. Squeezing them tightly, he acted as if he was trying to hold onto the mommy I was right in that moment, afraid that at any second I would change back to a screaming banshee.

We sat on the floor together, surrounded by a thousand Lego blocks. I tried to remember all the fun games we used to play at cleanup time. "Ready for basketball? Let's see who can throw the most pieces in the bucket the fastest."

"Okay, Mommy. I'm gonna win!"

For the next two years, I fought the same war, becoming severely depressed from constantly being told there was nothing wrong. I began to wonder if I needed drugs, a straitjacket, or worse, a lobotomy. Then it all came to a head in our local Target.

The kids and I had enjoyed a pleasant adventure surveying every aisle in the huge department store. I'd promised myself I would get through the outing without an angry or frustrated word.

"Kids, it's time to go home now," I said, in a rare composed manner.

Christmas was just around the corner, and we'd spent the last hour in the toy department taking notes on what to add to the list.

Even though it was a busy Tuesday afternoon, only two check stands were open. I knew we were in for a long wait, and began deep breathing for composure.

There I stood, clinging to the word "patient" in my mind, with my cart filled and four antsy kids. Timmy was in the basket seat, Jenni was hanging off the side, Lauren was hiding among the purchases, and Michelle was two steps ahead. Twenty minutes later, the check stand to the right opened up.

"Next person in line, please."

"Thank God! That's us, kids."

Carefully maneuvering my cumbersome load across the aisle to the right, I was almost run over by a hunchbacked elderly woman on a mission to get there first. Aggressively angling her way to the front, she began to take items out of her cart and place them on the counter.

"Excuse me," I said, politely. "I'm the next person in line."

The woman looked through her wire-rimmed granny glasses, peering down her long, skinny nose. She rolled her eyes and went back to her business.

"*Excuse me*," I said again, this time not quite as graciously. "It's the next person in line, and that's me!"

Again, she acted as if I wasn't even there and carried on unloading her purchases.

My blood began to boil, my hair stood on end, and venom seeped to the tip of my tongue. I didn't want to create a shouting match.

Instead, I pushed her aside and swept all her one-dollar shopper's specials back into her cart. Yanking the basket out of the lane, I thrust my mine in its rightful place.

"How rude!" the woman hissed to the multitude of shoppers waiting their turn.

That does it! I thought. Unable to hold my tongue any longer, I whipped around, my eyes bugging out of their sockets and arms in the air as if ready for a fight.

"Rude? You're calling *me* rude? Listen, lady, I've been standing here for an eternity with all these kids, and you butted in front of me. I think *you're* the one who's rude." Turning around, I looked at the checker, and asked calmly, "How much do I owe?"

The middle-aged, red-vested Target employee looked at me as if I was holding a knife in my hand and quickly told me my amount. Out the door I went with my horrified children.

"Mommy, are you okay?" Jenni asked, tears pouring out of her eyes.

"Sure, honey. I'm fine. Why do you ask?"

"You just screamed at that old lady."

"I did?" I wanted to act as if nothing had happened.

"Yeah. You've always told us to be nice to old people no matter what they do."

Realizing I had just performed a cardinal sin, I began to have a meltdown. Herding my crying kids into the car, I immediately pulled out my cell phone to call the doctor.

"I'll not take 'there's nothing wrong with you' for an answer any longer," I demanded. "I'm coming right over. You better make room for me."

After dropping the kids off at a neighbor's house, I found myself waiting in the examining room for the results of the blood test.

"Oh my God, Jackie," the doctor said. "You have absolutely no estrogen left in your body."

"Huh?"

"You're in menopause. We need to get you on some hormones."

"What? How can that be?" I cried.

"It's rare, but some women go through it early. Don't worry. It's not life threatening."

"Not for you. You don't live with me."

My doctor handed me pamphlet after pamphlet describing ways

to re-create what nature was prematurely taking away. There was the homeopathic method, the natural way through diet and organic foods, or the drug-induced scheme. Remembering what my mother had gone through—the rages, the tears, and the debilitating depression—I knew there was only one course of action to take.

"Just give me the damn drugs," I cried, disgusted at the untimely disintegration of my ovaries. "I don't have time to fool around with this any longer." I needed to get back to normal before my whole family ran away and I was left all alone in the world.

Driving home, reality slapped me across the face. At only forty years old, I was all dried up. There'd be no more babies. I'd turn lumpy and dumpy like so many other postmenopausal women. Wrinkles would begin to creep over my face, overemphasizing the road map of my life. I was doomed to become just like that old woman in Target.

Tears filled my eyes and soaked my cheeks until I could barely see the road ahead. I was having the pity party to end all parties. How could this be happening to me? I was too young.

"I hate you, God! This isn't fair," I shouted, realizing my dream for at least two more babies was squashed. "I'm not done."

Later that evening, I hid in my bedroom for fear I'd tear the head off of an unsuspecting family member. My children were now terrified of me, and I knew it would be days before the drugs kicked in. The best plan was to hole up.

Just as I was about to climb into my bed and sleep off the day, a barely audible tap sounded at the door. "Mommy," my five-year-old, Lauren, called softly. "Can I come in?"

"Are you sure you want to?"

Lauren's mahogany-colored eyes surveyed the room to make sure it was safe before she slowly tiptoed to my side.

"Mommy, I want you to feel better," she murmured in my ear, as she leaned in close to kiss my cheek.

Gathering her tiny body into my arms, I pulled her into the bed like I had so many other times in the middle of the night when she'd had a bad dream. Snuggling with her, I began to realize how blessed I was to have my children. Having babies was the one thing in my life that made me feel successful. But was it really important to have an army? What I already had was perfection.

"Honey, I'm sorry I've been so crabby. My body isn't working right, but the doctor thinks he can help me." Lightly planting soft butterfly kisses on her precious face, I tried to reassure her. "I hope you know how much I love you."

"I know, Mommy. Don't worry about the creepy old lady today in the store," Lauren rubbed her tiny nose across mine. "She was a real poop."

Soon the array of drugs (estrogen, progesterone, testosterone, and Prozac) began to kick in and I returned to normal—a little hazy, but alive and functioning. No longer did I freak out over the dirt children leave behind. I made sure I was always kind to the elderly, no matter how cranky they were, and I allowed Dave to do whatever he wanted, which included even more "boys' trips" away from the home and me.

The guilt left behind from my "bitch ordeal" made me want to please everyone nonstop. I fell deeper into a role of self-sacrifice and martyrdom to make up for all the wrongs I'd committed during those two horrible years.

What I didn't realize was that I was setting myself up for a gigantic fall, one I was totally unprepared for. It would take me years to unravel all that I'd set into motion.

Zookeeper

Raising children is a magical and daunting feat all in one. Magical when they turn into productive members of society; daunting when you wonder if they ever will. While they were little, I was the drill sergeant controlling their every action, thought, and food intake. When they became teenagers, they defied any form of adult manipulation and lost all the manners I had so diligently slaved to teach them.

"You are not the child I raised!" I constantly found myself screaming. "I taught you better than to talk like that! And what the hell are you saying anyway?" Often, I couldn't tell if the slang they used was inappropriate or not.

In the early years, I tried to set a pretty table: forks, knives, spoons, napkins, and a flower centerpiece. Somehow, the protocol I was imparting was just a futile attempt at teaching good etiquette. Rather than looking like genteel human beings, my children looked like a piglet family: rooting for food, snouts low, and grunting. The thought *How did I fail?* ran constantly through my mind.

"Mom, who cares how the food gets in my mouth as long as I clean my plate? Licking works great," Tim loved to inform me.

Day after day during those formative months when children are supposed to become adults and learn to take care of their personal needs,

I felt as if I was the warden of a zoo where deranged animals no other park would take were sent for display.

"Lauren, get out of that tree and stop throwing water balloons into the neighbor's yard." As I stood at the kitchen window, I could see my child dangling from the highest bough. "And, Tim, stop jumping off the roof onto the trampoline. You're going to hurt yourself."

"Oh, *Mom,*" they sang out in unison.

It was a day just like any other. As I passed each child's room, I was reminded that my home felt like a warehouse of cages. In each cage, a different animal waited for its escape, with a distinct odor all too indicative of the child that resided within.

"Oh my God! What's that stench, Michelle?" I was dismayed. After spending the entire morning cleaning, somehow chaos had reared its ugly head again, shortly after the three o'clock dismissal from school.

"It's the latest fragrance from Calvin Klein. Don't you just love it?" As she became lost in the foggy mist she was spraying all over her body, my fifteen-year-old daughter asked, "I also have Sunflower and Happy on. I wasn't sure which one to wear. What do you think?"

What do I think? I think I can't breathe.

"Ah, honey, it may be a little much," I responded, trying to be diplomatic. I knew if I didn't choose my words carefully, she'd do the exact opposite of what I wanted. "It would be more pleasant to the people around you if you just picked one fragrance at a time. How about baby powder? That has a nice, clean smell."

"Mom! You're so stupid." Michelle closed her door in my face. "No one wears baby powder."

I noticed a thick aroma coming from Jenni's room as well. "Have you been lending your perfumes to Jenni?"

"No!" Michelle flew out to investigate. "She better not be sneaking mine!"

"I'm sure she's not. It must be mine she's using." I knew I'd better cease and desist before I said something else that could cause World War III. I made a quick exit.

My first two girls were in their early teens. When they weren't dancing or rolling around in the mud playing sports, they were exploring their feminine sides. There were lotions, potions, and accessories that needed to be investigated.

My third daughter, on the other hand, preferred to live in squalor.

"My God, Lauren, this is gross!" I screamed, picking up her mud-covered soccer jersey.

"Mom, stop being so dramatic." Lauren threw her shin guards into the mix.

Lauren was always the athletic mammal in the group. Name the sport, and she played it with all the passion of a tiger looking for its next meal after a week of starvation.

"Lauren, I know you love to participate in every sport ever created, but you need to put your dirty clothes in the laundry room. Just look at this mess!" I gingerly picked up each item, as if it harbored some kind of rare disease. "You have your wet, grungy field hockey clothes rolled into a ball on top of your basketball jersey and volleyball uniform."

"They're not that bad," she replied casually. "You should see the other kids' clothes. This is nothing."

The worst offender to my delicate senses was my son. His room smelled like the local dump after a day or two of baking in one-hundred-degree heat. I was sure there must be a dead animal hidden under the piles of decomposing food, paper wrappers, smelly socks, and damp towels.

"Tim, you could have mold growing in this stuff," I scolded, looking at the mound before me. "Do you have any idea how poisonous that is?"

"Mom, you are so weird. Who cares? Besides, guys are supposed to be slobs."

"Tim, don't give me that 'this is what guys do' line. That's not an excuse for living in a pigsty. You are not some homeless animal living on nature's mercy." I chucked his laundry out of the room. "Get rid of the rotten food or, before you know it, that pet rat you've always wanted will bring its whole family to stay. But they won't be living in any cage."

Since it felt as if we lived in a zoo, I decided we might as well have some real animals to go with it. I'd heard that children who learn to care for a pet receive invaluable training on how to treat people. We started the long progression of creatures with the nondescript goldfish.

"Jenni, you need to feed the fish every day. You're their custodian, and without you they'll die."

"Okay, Mommy, I can do that, but will you help me wash the bowl?"

"Sure, honey."

Unfortunately, I was never good at rinsing any dish or glass object completely free of soap. Helpful Heloise I was not. Plus, I hated those boring, slimy creatures that spent their life swimming in only one direction, and always in circles. Once in a while, my lack of cleaning skills worked to my advantage.

Uh oh. I must not have washed the bowl very well. All the fish are floating at the top. Maybe if I flush them down the toilet and don't say anything, she'll forget we ever had them.

Our house became a domicile for birds, hamsters, guinea pigs, mice, chickens, carpenter ants, worms, bugs, and dogs. As I think back on that chaotic time in our lives, I find it funny how many of those creatures resembled my children in their various stages of development.

The rodents had a way of escaping their secure metal walls, just as my kids found ways to crawl out of the house late at night to meet up with their friends when I was fast asleep. Unlike those vermin, my sweet children would return to their individual pens and tuck themselves securely back in bed. I was never the wiser.

The egg-laying, two-legged feathered creatures were filthy, especially when they molted their feathers and left their droppings everywhere. In their own way, my kids were no different.

"Pick up this junk!" I hollered at yet another after-school disaster strewn all over the house. "You don't live in a cage that is self-contained. I have to live here too, you know. And while you're at it, someone flush the toilet!"

"Mom, I don't get you," Jenni yelled, running to the bathroom. "One minute you want us to throw our wet towels in the hamper, and the next you want us to hang them up to dry. Now it's all about flushing. I thought we were in a drought."

Not only do children come with messes, they also come with busy schedules. Until they were driving age, I would load up our green Suburban and shuffle them around, until I put over fifty miles on the car each day.

"Let's see. Lauren, your softball game starts at ten o'clock, and Jenni, yours at eleven. Michelle, you need to be at the dance competition at eight this morning, and Tim, you have baseball at twelve o'clock," I called out, as I threw breakfast on the table. But, unfortunately, it was never that easy.

Wait, where am I going? Is it Timmy at eight o'clock and Michelle at nine? Is Lauren dancing or playing basketball? I think I'm losing it.

I felt it was crucial that my kids know they had at least one parent in the stands, either cheering them on to victory or ready to wipe away tears that might come with the agony of defeat. Dave's increasingly busy schedule of golf trips (that he claimed were for business) kept him away for several days at a time. I was left alone with the task of making sure everyone got where they needed to go safely, in the correct (and clean) uniform, and on time.

"Okay, Jenni, you have a softball game in the North Bay. Tim, you have baseball in Sunnyvale. Michelle, you're competing somewhere near Sacramento, and Lauren, you have volleyball in East Jesus."

I didn't really just say that, did I?

As my brood became older, their powers of mother manipulation became increasingly more sophisticated. They learned the art of pestering, begging, and promising greatness if I'd succumb to their latest whim or desire.

"If you let me have this massive rager (teenage lingo for an out-of-control party), I promise no cops will come and I'll clean up everything."

"No, absolutely not," I growled at Michelle, now seventeen. "I will not be held responsible for anyone's illegal behavior. It'll get them a 'minor in possession' charge and land me in jail."

"God, Mom!" she bawled, stomping up the stairs. "That's not going to happen."

"You're right, it won't, because I'm not taking any chances."

Throughout those years, the Haugh house became home to not only my children, but the entire town of Los Altos. With four kids and at least ten extra friends per child on any given day (do the math: four times ten makes forty, plus my own kids for a total of forty-four), my home often felt like a boiling pot of hot water that was about to not just bubble over, but combust at any given moment. We became the party house, the gathering place for the group school project, the victory palace after sporting events (whether we won or lost) and in later years, the flophouse.

Oh my God! There must be twenty sleeping bodies piled on top of each other upstairs.

I ran into bedrooms, nudging my children's dead-to-the-world bodies. "Wake up, kids! Whose friends are these? Tell them it's time to go home. This is not the safe house for all the town drunks."

"Mom, can I tell them later?" Jenni asked in a groggy whisper, pulling the covers back over her face. "I'm too tired to get up. I'm going back to sleep."

The reality was that my house was a protected environment for kids to come to, and everyone knew it. Drinking or drugs were not allowed within the confines of my fortress, but no child was sent out into the night after a wild party elsewhere to drive under the influence, an act that could ruin their future or end their lives.

Ten years later, my little furry cubs have left the den and I'm left with an immaculate and peaceful playground. The cages have been disinfected. The doors are locked late at night, not to keep children in but invaders out. The stillness is deafening.

During those years of anarchy and constant bedlam, I clung to my daily sacred ritual, my evening bath, and prayed for the day when there would be peace and harmony in my life. Being able to concentrate only on my personal needs was a fantasy I held tight.

Won't it be heaven to just think about myself? It'll be paradise when the only laundry I'm responsible for is my own. And who will care if there's milk in the refrigerator?

Now, as I look around at my long-awaited paradise, I'm not so sure I like it. For twenty-seven years, I was a mother. For twenty-seven years, I was responsible for four human beings—their needs, their emotions, and their dreams. How do you find purpose in your life when the most important people are no longer there?

As I clean my house, I find myself wondering. *Where did it all go?* It was only yesterday when I fell into bed every night and passed out from physical, emotional, and mental exhaustion from trying to keep up with everyone. Now, my aging body keeps me awake with night sweats. There's no baby close by to help lull me to sleep.

As I lie alone in my California king-size bed in my empty house, I question how I'm supposed to sleep at all if I don't have someone's problem to solve. Despite the fact that the kids are scattered to the wind, I'm sure that in some sense they must need me. Staring at their pictures on the walls, a tear finds its way down my face. I know I still need them.

Sadie, Sadie, Married Lady

In my youth, my favorite daydream was finding that one special person who'd love me forever. Like many little girls, I was sure my handsome prince would one day swoop me off my feet and carry me away on his dazzling white stallion to a small cottage in the woods with a white picket fence. In the confines of our ideal world, I'd set up housekeeping as ten beautiful children ran naked and free. Together, we'd all live happily ever after. It would be years later that I discovered that the real-life story of my fairy tale marriage would unfold quite differently.

My children's father bulldozed his way into my life in the summer of 1978. I was twenty-five; he was twenty-two, and right out of Stanford University. He was brash, arrogant, brilliant, and the funniest person I'd ever met.

I was working for Century 21 Real Estate. Eyeing my future husband as I headed for my job on a rare warm June day in San Francisco, I wondered if we'd ever have the chance to actually meet. As the herd of cattle in their business attire squeezed together through the enormous steel doors of the Embarcadero Center elevator, Dave worked the morning crowd with his friendly manner and infectious personality. Telling jokes, laughing at the punch lines, and patting his neighbors on the back, he was young, tan, and handsome in his blue suit. By the time Dave reached his destination on the twenty-third floor, he had a pack of new best friends.

"I can't believe it," I said breathlessly, as I walked into my office that morning. "I saw the cutest guy on the elevator."

"Did you get his name?" Terri, the office manager, asked.

"No. And I'll probably never see him again."

Our building was one of the tallest high rises in the city in the mid-1970s. Because thousands of people came and went every day, hardly any ever crossed paths more than once every few years. Like ants dressed in polyester double knit suits, platform shoes, and very short skirts making their way through an ant farm, they walked single file to their destinations, eyes burrowing into the space straight ahead, and never looking sideways to acknowledge a coworker.

To my surprise, two days later Dave entered my office, clipboard in hand, and began asking the receptionist questions about our company's lease agreement.

"Jackie, can you help this guy?" the receptionist inquired, peeking around my door. "I've no idea what he's talking about."

With my heart in my throat, desperately trying not to release the butterflies that were about to flit out of my stomach, I extended my hand and guided Dave into the vice president's office. I didn't understand what he was asking either and felt that he should speak with the expert.

Upon leaving, he nonchalantly stopped at my desk to chat.

I can't believe this guy is actually in my office, I thought as I watched his animated face and listened to him ramble. Within seconds, he began to try to make arrangements for our first lunch date.

"Want to go to lunch today?" he asked warmly, his charismatic smile gleaming.

"I'm sorry, I can't today," I answered, playing hard to get. I had never wanted a date so badly, but I loved watching him work at getting me to say yes.

"How about tomorrow?"

"Sorry."

After giving Dave the same answer for every day in the week, I finally consented to the following Friday. That would give me a week to start preparing for the meal that would steer me off the road I was currently traveling and change my life forever. I'd always been attracted to the sweet and unassuming type of male who was as humble as he was kind. Dave couldn't have been more different.

At six feet tall, his strong athletic build, obsidian eyes, and contagious laugh were the finishing touches to the confidence that oozed from every pore in his body. He was a man with direction, purpose, and determination to get what he wanted. There'd be no stopping him on his mission. I was totally enamored.

Unfortunately, the day for which I had set such high expectations was less than exhilarating. On the date, I quickly became unimpressed with the other side of Dave's personality.

"Waitress, take this back," he demanded in an icy tone.

"What's wrong with your food?" I asked, since it looked perfectly fine to me.

"I asked for it medium rare," he stated. "It's more medium and I want it right."

"Is it really that big of a deal?" Never in my life had I sent something back to a kitchen. I was always so glad just to be able to go out in the first place. Anything would have been fine.

"You pay for service too. If the service is lousy, I don't leave a good tip."

As Dave delved further into his conversation, I found him to have an egotistical manner. He made crude remarks about the waitress and other patrons in the restaurant, all topped by an obnoxious demeanor I found insufferable. We had nothing in common, and I couldn't wait for the meal to be over.

After an hour of Dave's monopolizing the entire conversation as I nodded to be polite, I decided to participate in his long-winded conversation. I needed to hear the sound of my own voice for some sanity.

"What exactly is your job with Coldwell Banker? Are you a survey man or what?" I asked coldly. I was remembering how my boss had come out of his office and questioned, "Who was that guy?" We already had our lease locked in with Coldwell Banker for fifteen years. Dave was a new intern with this prestigious real estate firm, and the questions he'd asked had been highly irregular.

Leaning back in his chair, he gave a smug smile that lit up his whole face, as if to say *Gotcha*. "Do you really want to know?"

Is this some type of trick question? I wondered. "Yes, I want to know."

"I had to find a way to meet you," Dave began. "When I saw you in the elevator, I knew you were someone I wanted to get to know." As he leaned forward, his overly self-confident manner began to soften. "I told the guys in the office about my dilemma, so my boss handed me his clipboard and told me to pretend I was analyzing the building and the existing leases."

Stunned, I asked, "How'd you know where to find me?"

"I saw you push twenty-seven. When I got off the elevator, I went to every tenant." Dave chuckled. "Your office was the last one, but by then I had my spiel down good."

Overly aggressive men had pursued me before, but Dave took the prize. As his gentler side surfaced, I could see that his boldness during the meal was perhaps a nervous attempt to make a good impression. Behind all his hoopla, there was an interesting, and obviously creative, person. Instantly I thought he deserved another chance.

Three months later, we were engaged to be married.

Unfortunately, the first several years of our marriage were not the honeymoon bliss I expected. Being three years older, I was done with college antics and was ready to settle down for a family life. Dave, on the other hand, would forever be a highly spirited, fun-loving, magical character: Peter Pan. But instead of living in never-never land, he'd keep one foot firmly planted in his old frat *Animal House* lifestyle.

"Who are all these guys?" I asked as I came in from the grocery store. Shirtless, inebriated men were strewn all over our living room, whooping and hollering at the television.

"Just a few of my buddies to watch the game. Would you make us something to eat?"

We were living in San Diego at the time, and I didn't have a soul to call my friend. It was Dave's hometown. His entire family lived there, as well as his childhood cronies. I was completely alone and desperately wanted and needed my husband's attention. But I seemed to be constantly nudged aside. I didn't realize the fun aspect of his personality that I loved so much in the engagement period would have to be shared with the world once we were married.

Every weekend, our home seemed to be the playground for all the big boys to hang out. It also became my responsibility to see that they were well fed and lubricated with a well-stocked refrigerator.

"What do you guys want?" I sighed, knowing I was in for a long and loud afternoon.

"Sandwiches. Oh, and bring that twelve pack of Coors over too," Dave yelled above the football game. "We just finished this one."

A few years later, after all four of the children were born, Dave's need to play with the boys kept him away not only during the daytime, but later into the evenings. Lying in bed, I would watch the hands of the clock tick into the early morning hours. Cell phones had not yet become a household staple, and like the mother of a teenager who'd just gotten his license, I panicked as I prayed that he'd come home safe.

"Dave, do you know what time it is?" I asked groggily, watching him tiptoe in at three in the morning.

"Sorry, I guess time got away from me."

"Got away from you? What the hell were you doing?" I demanded, realizing Timmy's four o'clock feeding was around the corner.

"We were only playing cards and drinking. Nothing to worry about."

Those words, "nothing to worry about," would become prophetic, and something I should have paid closer attention to.

In the early days of raising children, I was surrounded by constant bedlam. It took every ounce of energy I had to keep things running smoothly. Strangers often asked me, "How many children do you have?"

"Five," I'd giggle. "My husband is the oldest."

Over the years, childrearing and menopause took their toll on me. I was beyond exhausted. It was bad enough trying to keep up with teenagers, but I couldn't keep up with my oldest frenetic "child" either.

"Come on, Jack," Dave said, when he saw me passed out one evening. "Let's get out. Every night I come home you're flaked out on the bed."

I wondered why he couldn't understand how difficult my days were. "I'm sorry, Dave. Today was horrible. This morning I had to take Mom to her doctor's appointment. Then I taught three hours of dance and spent the afternoon driving the kids around, all while dealing with their emotional issues. I can't move."

"Fine. Just lay there, but I'm going out!"

I watched him pick up his keys again and head for the door. I knew I should jump off the bed, pull myself together, and join him, but my desire to please and be the good wife was being squashed with another budding migraine headache. To top it off, there was that sick feeling deep inside that he really didn't want me anyway.

Why bother? I know if I go, he won't pay any attention to me.

I wiped the tears that were pooling in my eyes. The thought of being left in a corner all night by myself was more than I could handle.

Marriage is a balance of give and take. I gave and Dave took. I wanted to please, so any needs I had were put on the back burner and I decided to rarely fight with him. The little hippie girl from the early 1970s, extolling the virtues of "make love not war," rose again from the ashes. But instead of resembling the Phoenix, the strong and powerful Greek bird that symbolizes rebirth, I looked more like a battered seagull that had barely made it to shore from the hurricane brewing at sea. I was in a constant state of warfare with the kids. I couldn't handle one more battle at the end of the day with my life partner.

"Jackie, if I ran my business like you run this house we'd be broke," Dave told me one night.

"I'm doing the best I can." I could hear how uncertain I sounded. "Why is it so important that the house be clean all the time?"

"You have the time. You're home all day," he grunted, sitting down to watch the TV. "You Los Altos housewives have it so easy."

I wondered: *How could you possibly know how easy I have it? You're hardly ever here.* I was afraid to get into a verbal battle of wits. I instinctively knew I would lose. Dave had an answer for everything. Quietly, and dutifully, I began the never-ending cleanup.

It's been said that bad things happen to good people. In our case, a good person decided to do a bad thing. Dave rolled twenty-two years of marriage up into a paper ball and threw it into the trashcan, like an insignificant piece of scribble with words that no longer made sense. He became unhappy with his wife and the life we shared. I was boring, uninspiring, and paid too much attention to the children. My husband felt lonely and unappreciated and went elsewhere to look for his "fun and passion." What better place than with the younger assistant at the office?

"I can't believe he'd leave," I sobbed to the therapist. "Not after all I did and the freedom I gave him."

Angry thoughts of the endless nights I'd stayed home alone while he was out playing deluged my aching heart. What a fool I'd been. From the early days of my expulsion from Miss Nancy's School of Dance, I'd committed myself to being the good girl, the pleaser, and where did it get me? Alone.

Divorce hammered me through the typical progression of grief, anger, loss, loneliness, and gut-wrenching trepidation. For me, it also went a step deeper. My world was forcefully pulled apart and shredded in the garbage disposal. A promise was broken, but more importantly, so was my lifelong dream.

"I don't think I'll ever be able to trust anyone again." My voice cracked. I'd been seeing Dr. Grey for over a year, and the healing process was still eluding me.

"Jackie, you will, but it takes time."

"I'm just so angry. I actually think I hate him," I muttered, twisting a wad of Kleenex to shreds. "I can't seem to move forward. I feel like I'm constantly being shoved against a wall."

With a kind and wise smile, Dr. Grey took my hand. "You need to learn to forgive, and then you can move on."

Shocked at her suggestion, I just stared at her. She knew all the dirty details of the day-in and day-out divorce proceedings. It was a constant battle over the kids and money. I wanted to vomit every time I heard Dave's voice on the phone.

"Jackie, forgiveness is a gift you give yourself. It's not for Dave's benefit. He doesn't care if you forgive him or not." Sitting back in her chair, Dr. Grey took a breath and continued, "It's only when you let go of the hurt and anger that you will learn to trust again."

Driving home that cold winter's afternoon, I watched as the sun slipped behind massive cumulus clouds. As the heavens lit up with brilliant shades of red, pink, and purple, I thought God was letting me know, in His usual quiet manner, that He was there to help me. He was also whispering that I had another job to do. I had to add "peacemaker" to my long list of duties.

Arriving home, I went straight to the place that helped me see things clearly when I felt lost. I climbed out Michelle's bedroom window, sat on the roof with my knees tucked to my chest, and watched the last of the miraculous spectacle unfold in the western sky.

How do I even begin to forgive? This was not part of the vision.

I wanted to blame Dave, and Dave alone, for what I felt was the destruction of a lifelong quest for ultimate happiness. It *had* to be his fault. I was loyal. I was faithful. I'd played the game and followed all the rules. But the nagging little voice of reason that tickled my conscience told me something different: maybe I was to blame, too.

When Dave and I first met, I was at a low point in my life and stunted in my emotional growth. Two years earlier, I had found the type of man I always hoped would be in my life. Shaun resembled a large teddy bear, rounded at the middle with an already thinning hairline. He was gentle and kind and was all about me and my needs, or so I thought.

"What do you mean you're leaving?" I cried, the night he shocked me with the news he was moving back to Los Angeles to be with his high school sweetheart.

"Sorry, Jackie," Shaun answered, his eyes never making contact with mine.

"So, was all that talk about our getting married a lie?"

"Sorry." And with that, he walked out of my life, leaving me feeling that I'd never be good enough for anyone. The way I figured it, if a "good guy" like Shaun didn't want me, who would?

In that coming-of-age period when I was twenty-three, I kept all my fears, hurts, and pain locked away from the world. Other than a blank stare that occasionally crossed my face when I was most terrified, no one ever knew what I was thinking or feeling, especially at work.

"Jackie, get in here," my boss yelled a few weeks after the breakup.

"Yes?"

"What is wrong with you?" she demanded, holding up a stack of papers marked with erratic scratches of red pen. "Each one of these entries is a mess. I asked you to proof them. Have you even looked at them?"

Choking up, I held my hand in a tight fist, hoping the strength in my fingers would keep me from bursting into a tsunami of tears. "I—"

"You what?" my boss snarled. She threw the stack on her desk, papers flying in all directions.

Silence.

And then it happened. The story I'd hidden from the world for the past several weeks, of my first true love abandoning me for another woman, poured from my sobbing body. For ten minutes, the tale of love found and lost spewed from me. As my story came to an end, my usually tough and unsympathetic boss stood up, put her arms around me, and told me to go home for the rest of the day.

"Jackie, get some sleep," she said, opening the door to her office. "You look like hell. Tomorrow will be better."

"You're not firing me?"

"No. I think you've already been fired." She smiled. "I'm here to give you another chance. But first, you get some rest."

Sitting on the San Francisco bus that foggy afternoon, I made a vow to myself. For weeks I'd lived in the bottom of a dank well with no way to climb out. But from that day forward, I promised I'd never let anyone hurt me that deeply again. Scaling out of my circular hell, I would become determined to build a strong fortress, brick by brick, around my heart.

Just as I'd finally given up on the idea of ever meeting someone, Dave blasted into my world and threw me into the front seat of his roller coaster. He wasn't the type of man I thought I'd ever marry, but I did know he was a decent human being, despite the wild bravado. He had the confidence that our union was the right move, and I let him believe for both of us. The one dream we shared was a life with lots of kids. Since I felt I'd never find a soulmate, my new quest had become to find a wonderful father for my unborn children.

Time has a way of keeping a Band-Aid on the sore until it's ripped off. The wound may still be visible, but the excruciating pain is gone. When my Band-Aid was removed after the divorce, friends asked me, "Why did you ever marry him in the first place?"

"I had my reasons." Thinking of my children, I added: "Besides, just look at what I got! I'd do it all over again."

The period after the legal papers were signed was brutal for my children, as well as for me, and the recovery took several years. But anger was too exhausting an emotion to harbor. Gradually, the children made their peace with their father, with my guidance.

"Kids, you have to remember your dad loves you," I reminded them constantly. "You need to have him in your life."

"Mom, I don't get how you and Dad ever got together," Jenni said one day, during a rare visit home during her spring break from the University of Arizona. "You two are so different."

Remembering how she'd been the one child who desperately wanted us to stay married, I giggled that she could now see us for who we really were.

"Honey, I truly believe your father and I were meant to be together," I said, giving her a quick hug. "Yes, we're very different, but when you kids were little, we worked well together and we wanted the same thing: a home with a family. You really got the best from both of us. I taught you your morals and spiritual values, and he taught you how to have fun in life."

I was reminded of all Dave gave to me too. Besides four wonderful children, he gave me the gift of being a stay-at-home mom when they were little. After he left, I grew to appreciate the pressure he must have been under during the difficult times when the money wasn't flowing. It's no wonder he thought my life looked easy.

Thinking back to our early years, I knew I needed to remember that it hadn't been all bad. It's very easy to forget the good when the heart is shrouded in tremendous pain. By three years after Timmy was born, I'd actually felt that perhaps Dave did love me. Maybe not the way I needed to be loved, but in his own way, he cared. We'd been happy and enjoyed each other's company.

The one thing I never doubted was his love for his children. Until he lost his way, he'd been the father I always dreamed I wanted for my kids, entertaining and hands-on.

Time heals all wounds. For me, it helped me see that my heart wasn't really broken with the dissolution of our twenty-two years together. How could it be broken if it was never completely given in the first place? I loved Dave, but I'd never fully permitted him into my soul, and for that I was to blame. I'd been fearful I'd be criticized or told that I was stupid. We'd never spoken the same emotional language. The thought of rejection over my thoughts and dreams helped to keep the brick wall up around my heart permanently.

Instead of discussing with my husband the vital issues that made me tick as a woman, I turned to the diaries I was keeping for my children to let that voice be heard. Fearful I might die when they were young, and that their father would never be able to fully describe me, I wanted something left behind to help them know and understand the woman who'd carried them inside her belly. The woman who adored them more than life itself.

Instead of a heart, a dream was broken: the dream of being together and watching our children have children. The dream of rediscovering the person I married in our later years and growing old together. The dream of security. Fortunately, dreams can be rebuilt.

Today, eight years later, Dave and I are friends. It wasn't easy, but I took Dr. Grey's advice and forgave him for what I felt were selfish actions. It's incredible how freeing forgiveness can be. We'll always be connected through our four children, and I want that union to be harmonious. There will be graduations, weddings, and future grandchildren that we must share. Being hateful only hurts the one who is hating.

Now that I've moved to the next phase of my life, I plan to tear down all those internal barriers that I set up years before. Walls not only keep others out, but hold me locked inside. I want to free myself to fresh possibilities and create new dreams with the person I know will be that soulmate: that special person perfectly created by the universe meant just for me. I'm sure he's out there waiting.

Bewitched

My fiftieth birthday was just around the corner, and the roles of parent and child had reversed. As if by magic, my children became responsible adults raising me, their broken mother who had completely lost her way.

Getting out there, as my children called it, had been hard enough when I was in my early twenties. But as I approached the half-century mark, it was pure torture. Looking into the mirror each morning reminded me that there was no turning back. There were wrinkles, sagging loose skin that drooped off my knees and elbows, jiggling inner thighs, and a sagging chest. Brown spots emerged on the backs of my hands. In my mouth, "long of tooth" reared its ugly head as the gums receded higher and higher into my jaw. Toothpicks became just as important to my daily beauty routine as an eyelash curler.

It was much easier to stay home, planted in front of the television set or curled up with a good book.

"Mom, you need to get out more," Tim, now fourteen, said every night over dinner.

"You just want to get rid of me," I replied, kissing his head. "I know you want to have a party."

"No, I mean it. I don't like seeing you sit home."

Michelle, by virtue of being the oldest, was the most experienced in life and made it her mission to find ways to help me live again. She had worked way too hard in high school teaching me how to dress and wear my makeup to keep me acceptable in the eyes of her friends. She was not about to see all her hard work go down the drain.

"Mom, come visit me," she would periodically implore, from her apartment near UCLA. "You need to get out of Los Altos and come play with me."

"Honey, I can't do that. I still have your brother and sister to take care of."

"Mom, there's such a thing as getting a babysitter or passing them off to their friends for a night," she chided. "Stop making excuses."

One Friday night, on a weekend visit home from college in her junior year, Michelle told me stories of her adventures with her friends and her latest part-time job working at the Playboy Mansion in Beverly Hills.

As I looked at her fresh, young face, giant blue eyes, and long, wavy blond hair, I couldn't get over our similarities at the same age. I'd had similar conversations with my own mother about the exploits of a busy college coed. It seemed like just yesterday.

"Is this a real job? I hope you have your clothes on."

"Oh God, Mom! Yeah, it's a real job." Michelle picked at the salad I was trying to finish making. "I wear a waitress outfit and serve at all the big parties. Next week they've asked me to work at some lame event. I don't think I want to go."

"What is it?"

"Some stupid astronauts will be there to celebrate a space writer."

"Who's the writer?" I inquired, knowing this would not be some dull event.

"A guy named Arthur Clarke. Supposedly he wrote *2001: A Space Odyssey*. They turned it into a movie." She sighed heavily. "I guess they named a robot after him that was sent to Mars."

In 2001, NASA had hurled a robotic spacecraft into the universe in a burning quest to find life in outer space. The importance of this mission was completely lost on my child.

I grabbed the salad before Michelle ate all the good stuff and left me only lettuce. "Sounds interesting to me. Do you know who else will be there?"

"I think they said Buzz Aldrin, Jim Lovell, and Neil Armstrong, plus a lot of movie stars who were in science fiction films or TV shows."

It was obvious to me that my daughter's early education had missed the important chapter on space exploration and what it meant. Back in 1969, when Neil Armstrong took the first step on the moon, I was sixteen. As I'd looked up at the heavens while sitting at a baseball game with my boyfriend, the knowledge that one of America's finest was roaming around on that brightly lit ball was the most exciting moment in the history of the world to me. What seemed to be an impossible feat had become a reality and taught me to believe that dreams really do come true with enough work and perseverance.

"Honey, they aren't just some guys. They're American heroes. You should go!"

"Sounds boring."

"Trust me. You should go. I would."

Jumping off the kitchen counter, Michelle sauntered off to the computer. Within a few minutes, she was back again, wearing a Cheshire cat smile from ear to ear.

"Mom, you need to make a plane reservation and come to L.A. next weekend. I got you a job at the mansion."

"*What?*" I was so shocked, I nearly slammed my finger in the dishwasher.

"I emailed my boss and said I'd do it only if you could too." She gave me a hug. "He asked what you looked like. I told him you were hot!"

"You told him I was hot?" I was amused that my twenty-year-old found her mother even the slightest bit attractive.

"I told him you were really, really hot, so he said, 'Bring her on!' No excuses this time. Find Timmy and Lauren a place to stay for the weekend."

A week later, I boarded Southwest Airlines for the first paid waitressing job of my life.

Standing in front of the hotel mirror as I prepared myself for the evening ahead, I surveyed the image before me. I smoothed down the seams of my white starched shirt, sleeveless and formfitting. As I brushed the lint from my tight black pants, a nervous smile crept over my face.

I hope I don't embarrass Michelle. How many mothers ever get an opportunity like this? I didn't want to blow it and have my child feel sorry she ever thought of the idea.

"You look perfect, Mom," Michelle said proudly, as I climbed into her Ford Explorer. "Chef is going to love you."

"Chef?"

"Yeah, that's what we call him. He's the boss."

Arriving at the mansion at five o'clock, we parked at the bottom of the hill leading to the long driveway with the other hired help.

"Michelle, couldn't we have gotten a little closer to the house? This walk is going to kill me," I grumbled, taking off my spiked high-heeled shoes.

"Mom, you're a server, not a guest. It's not much further. Why did you wear such fancy shoes?"

"I wanted to look good." Now I was feeling rather foolish. "It's not often a regular mom gets to go to the Playboy Mansion."

Walking onto the property, I felt as if I'd stepped into the Twilight Zone. I was struck with the opulence and decadence of Hugh Hefner's thirty-room Gothic-style mansion. Glass-paneled French doors opened into the lush garden, where flamingos pranced about in the early evening light. Heavy tan velvet curtains draped the windows, and through the opening I could see that the ceiling was covered in beautiful frescoes.

The kitchen, however, was another story. Built for the mass production of food, the counters and cabinetry were designed for function and not beauty. A bouquet of smells permeated the room. Warm bread was baking in the oven, while curry chicken simmered on the stove. On the side counter were a plethora of sweet desserts: white- and dark-chocolate-covered strawberries, lemon cheesecake, almond torte, and a massive mocha-cherry four-layer cake.

Events for the rich and famous were held on the grounds several times a week, so efficiency was not just necessary, but crucial.

As the cooks flew back and forth from the sinks to the refrigerator and pantries, two peroxide-blond, curvaceous "bunnies" came in for their late afternoon snack. Taking no notice of all the commotion, the buxom bombshells pilfered the hors d'oeuvres trays.

"Oh my God, Michelle. Look at the size of those breasts!" I whispered into my daughter's ear. "Two of mine wouldn't even begin to equal one of theirs."

"You know they're fake. Just like their personalities."

"I wonder how they move around with those big honking things?" I glanced down at the two measly mounds planted on my chest.

"Get your mind off boobs, Mom. It's time to work."

After meeting Chef, a middle-aged, gray-haired man of portly stature, we were told our duties. Since Michelle had worked there several times before (and she was drop-dead gorgeous), she was on the A-list for serving. I was on the B-list. It was Michelle's responsibility to pass appetizers and mingle with the guests. I had to wait in the wings until it was time for the buffet line, where I would schlep pumpkin ravioli.

"Honey, who's out there?" I asked, as Michelle ran by me to grab another tray. The cocktail hour ran from five to seven o'clock. Waiting to get my first glimpse of a star felt like an eternity.

"Tom Hanks and his wife, Rita," Michelle called out, making a quick U-turn back out again. "Oh, and a bunch of old guys from *Star Trek*."

"Those *old guys* happen to be close to *my* age!" I called out, but that failed to make an impression on my child.

While standing off to the side, trying not to get in anyone's way and keeping completely to myself, I watched in amazement how nimbly all the workers refilled the trays. Large silver platters of stuffed mushrooms, miniature quiches, and cheese croquettes circulated back and forth. Chef's kitchen was run with lightning-fast precision. Not one morsel of food ever dropped to the floor.

On Michelle's next visit to the kitchen, she shoved her loaded tray into my hands. "Here, Mom, get out there! Hurry before Chef sees you."

"Honey, I can't do that. I'll get fired."

"Mom, this is your chance to see what's happening out there. Who cares if he fires you? You're never coming back here anyway." Taking the orchid from her ear and sticking it behind mine, Michelle propelled me out the door to the crowd waiting by the pool.

It was a typical warm, eighty-degree November evening in Los Angeles, and the guests were dressed in their finest tuxedos and gowns. Across the yard, the distinguished men of honor stood in their aerospace uniforms, rows and rows of medals hanging from their breast pockets. The lines on their weathered faces told a story all by themselves. These gentlemen had seen things few could imagine existed. To the right of the pool was James Cameron, holding court with some blond, nipped-and-tucked Hollywood beauties. Swans floated in the water nearby.

Remember, they're just people, I kept repeating in my mind as I made my way to the patio.

"Excuse me, miss. Miss? May I try some?" a voice asked from behind. I turned around slowly, trying to keep my tray intact.

I was face-to-face with my favorite actor, Morgan Freeman!

"Ah, would you like some tuna tartar?" I suggested, trying to act nonchalant.

"Sure. Hey, Patrick, try these out."

Patrick Stewart of *Star Trek: The Next Generation* strolled over for several helpings. There we were—me, Morgan, and Patrick—conversing over some grated raw fish and the balmy weather.

I returned to the kitchen in disbelief, where I spotted my daughter. "Michelle, you'll never guess who I just talked to!"

"Oh God, Mom! I see famous people at these things all the time."

"But, honey—"

"Mom, I'm happy you're happy, but it's time to serve dinner."

Dinner was held in an enormous tent that seated close to two hundred and fifty people. An ice sculpture of a spaceship was the centerpiece. In each of the drinks were acrylic cubes that lit up in bright fluorescent red, green, and blue. Overhead, brilliant stars hung from the canopy. The crisp white linens fluttered in the evening breeze that wafted through the seams of the canvas.

Still hanging onto my short-lived starstruck moment, I made my way to the buffet line. I found myself spooning pasta with a creamy orange sauce out to the likes of Tom Paxton and Kathleen Quinlan of the movie *Apollo 13*, William Shatner and Leonard Nimoy of the original *Star Trek* series, and Hugh Hefner's two young sons.

"What is this slop?" Tom Paxton inquired, with a twinkle in his eyes.

"Some ravioli dish. I think it's supposed to be healthy," I quipped. "It's made from the pumpkins Hugh grows on his estate."

"Really?"

"Really. Didn't you know that he tends to plump, ripe vegetables as well as women?"

"Well, I hope it's better than the roast beef," Paxton whispered. "It looks like it's been circling the earth a few times before it landed here."

During my marriage, I was never good at small talk. In fact, I deplored trying to think of things to say to people I didn't know. My children's father constantly took me to large events, where he'd leave me alone while he worked the crowd. I found this to be cruel and unjust punishment.

But in this fairy tale moment, I somehow found my voice with ease and humor. I chatted with every person who came my way.

"So tell me, what's life like here in Hollywood?" I asked Kevin Bacon, one of the stars from *Apollo 13*. Considering that he was both famous and married to the beautiful Kyra Sedgwick, I was sure it was nothing but glamorous.

"Life here is like life anywhere," he responded nonchalantly. "We have kids that we're constantly running around after. We have the same needs to be loved as anyone else, and we all go the bathroom in the exact same manner. Hopefully, with the door closed." With a wink and a smile, he moved on.

At the end of the evening, walking down the steep hill to Michelle's car, I was on a high I'd never felt before. "No one is going to believe what I did tonight," I said, hugging my daughter.

"I'm glad you had a good time, Mom. But I'm so over all this. I don't think I want to do another one of these events."

I stopped dead in my tracks and turned to her. "You've got to be kidding me! I'd come back."

"Nope, you're done. Now it's time we try something else."

"Like what? What could be better than this?"

"You'll see."

For the next several years, "something else" meant my children accepting me as one of their gang. There was partying with my now-grown daughters Michelle and Jenni, shooting the breeze with Tim and his buddies, dancing whenever music was heard (even on tabletops), and eating at restaurants where we were sure to see movie stars.

My daughters and I even made trips to bars on the dark side, with pseudo-masochistic elements.

"Girls, I don't think I belong in here," I mumbled in horror, as I watched gaunt figures amble about the dank and oppressive room. The place resembled a dark cave where you could barely see your hand in front of your face, except with the help of a pocket cigarette lighter here and there. This was not your typical watering hole.

"Michelle, what's with these half-naked, bald women tied up in chains?"

As she guided me past a row of live mannequins shackled along the walls, Michelle informed me, "Oh, they're just decorations."

"Decorations? They look like they've been starved to death. I think it's time for me to leave."

"Oh, no you don't. Have a stiff drink and find the dance floor," Jenni commanded, taking my hand to the bar. "You are not some typical housewife. You were meant to explore."

And explore I did. My brood grabbed hold of me, yanked me out of the house, and taught me to try new things, mingle with the best and most depraved of life, and to do it all with a smile. I was also taught how to get out of any uncomfortable situation.

"Just leave the party if you're not having fun," Lauren told me, as I was preparing myself for yet another Los Altos party where I would be the only single woman there. "You've got your car. The main thing is that you at least try to get through the evening."

"But, honey, I'm afraid that would be rude. It's probably best if I just don't go."

"No! You need to go and stay as long as you can. Too bad if it looks rude," she encouraged. "You have to take care of yourself."

Hmm, take care of myself, I thought. *Now that's a new concept.*

Once my social graces improved, my guardian angels decided it was high time I found a man, but only one with potential. They were not about to let their mother become some pathetic old maid, but they were also not going to let her settle for just anyone.

"Mom, Kelly and I decided you and her father should go out together,"

Lauren announced one day as she came in from basketball practice. Kelly was an early childhood friend of Lauren's, and surrogate daughter to me. I had known her father from the days of grammar school softball games, where we coached against each other. As we were both single parents, our families together melded into one. I'd stepped in when his children needed a mom, and vice versa.

"Oh, honey, you've got to be kidding. He's like my brother."

"That's why it would be perfect. He's already part of the family," she stated proudly, as if she had discovered the cure to the common cold.

"Sorry, Lauren. That feels too incestuous."

"Can't you at least *think* about it?" she called out, as she walked to her bedroom.

Bending over to pick up the basketball shoes she'd left behind on the floor, I was reminded of all the times each one of my children had eyed a prospective candidate and tried to arrange a meeting.

Would that ever work? I wondered, knowing what a good catch Kelly's dad was. But then I thought better. *Oh my God! What am I thinking? We are so different in the way we approach life that we'd probably eat each other alive. It's best we stay just friends.*

Even though I was making great progress, I wondered if I'd ever be adult enough in my kids' eyes to make it on my own. Surrounded by strong, confident individuals, my kids quickly began to glue me, their Humpty Dumpty, back together. When I got too thin, they told me to eat more. When I got crabby or depressed, they told me it was time to take a nap. When I got scared about my new career in real estate, they expressed confidence in me. And, when I was in doubt about my parenting skills, they bolstered my ego.

"I'm so lucky to have you kids," I told fifteen-year-old Tim while we were having dinner together one night. All the girls were now grown and out of the house, and it was just my baby and me. "You've all been so wonderful."

"Mom, luck had nothing to do with it."

Looking up from my meal, I stared into the face of this man-child who'd always displayed more integrity than any adult male I'd ever known. "No, Tim, really. Think about your friends and the trouble they get themselves into. You kids have been so easy to raise."

"It's not about luck. We are who we are because of you." Looking straight into my eyes with conviction, he continued, "You've always given us enough rope to test the water, but you've never left us dangling when we needed help. You've created your own luck by always being there for us."

I'd like to think that my son's words are true, but the truth is that God blesses us all with gifts that enrich our lives. Those blessings may be a brilliant mind, physical strengths, or artistic abilities that create beautiful surroundings. My gifts are my children.

Because of the four of them, I knew I had a reason to live when dark, evil thoughts of ending it all entered my maimed emotions during my divorce. They made me feel worthy. They showed me how to take chances, discover new things, and leave my couch without being afraid. With their magic powers, and the grace of God, I became free, no longer afraid of my own shadow, ready to do what I put off for fifty years: live my own life.

The Neighborhood Specialist

The Bible says that the love of money is the root of all evil. Unfortunately, it was a wickedness I grew to love. During my twenty-two-year union with my children's father, I became the personification of an American consumer, molded by greed to devour all of life's unnecessary products.

As a baby boomer, I grew up in an era where success meant giving your children an education, having little discretionary cash for anything else. Never did I realize there was an electrifying world out there that money could buy. Raised with an overprotected view of the almighty dollar, my parents drilled that it should be spent only when necessary. Affluence during my life with Dave was unlike anything I'd ever known, and I was determined to never go back in time.

Little did I realize that when my marriage ended, so too would my frivolous lifestyle. With Dave's departure, so departed the funds to pay off the mountain of invoices that came in daily. By deciding to keep our family home and our cabin in Tahoe, I became property rich and cash poor. Not only did it become my responsibility to fix five broken hearts (as well as the broken furnace), it was now also my daunting duty to pay the bills.

Hmm, which piggy bank do I break into first? I sighed, looking at the stack of bills before me. *Let's see, I can pay the mortgage, the car payment, insurance, and taxes. I can pay the Visa bill for all the new clothes the kids need for school, and will have just enough left over for my nails.*

As I put all of life's necessities into neat little piles, I came to the conclusion that there had to be priorities for payment. Personal appearance and the tax man were far more crucial than nutrition, so back to hot dogs it would be until I found some forgotten money under the mattress.

"I'm sorry, kids," I apologized, as they looked into the empty refrigerator for the fifth day in a row. "I don't have extra money right now for snacks."

"Maybe if you stopped having your nails done, you would," Jenni sneered, slamming the cabinet door.

Looking at my long gel-filled French manicure, the only pretty thing left on my aging body, I mumbled, "No. I'll find some other way to feed you."

My first visit to a nail salon had occurred when Timmy was three. At that point, I no longer had to worry about the residue a dirty diaper might leave behind in the deep crevices of elongated acrylic tips. Having my nails done was a sign to the world that I had finally made it in society. I was a woman of leisure, who had a few extra bucks each week to fritter away on this shameful extravagance. Losing them would surely mean I was headed for the poorhouse.

But after two years of throwing the pieces of my financial life up in the air like a highly skilled juggler pitching and catching a twelve-pack of eggs, I realized I was going to have to get a real job. One of those horrible time-suckers whose only saving grace was a paycheck that came every two weeks. More income was a vital necessity, especially if I wanted nice-looking hands. Looking at bare and unpolished nails would be a daily reminder of what I had lost.

I mulled over my possibilities for employment. I thought about going back to school and becoming a classroom teacher. But who wanted to deal with parents who thought their child was the only perfect student in class and deserved your undivided attention for near poverty-level pay?

Then there was the makeup consultant job opening at Nordstrom. I always loved playing with cosmetics, and in my earlier days I was an artist. I had a good sense for color, but realized it would take supernatural feats to make women in their eighties look fifty again. I was having enough trouble concealing the wrinkles on my own face. Plus, that was also a minimum-wage job.

My father noticed the look of panic on my face as I sat down to pay the electric bill. "Jackie, let me put together a budget for you," he suggested. A math genius, my dad was a whiz at keeping our family ledger balanced, a trait his daughter never inherited.

A budget! Oh God, not one of those.

"Thanks for the offer, Dad," I said, kissing him on the cheek, "but I'll figure this out."

After the tossing and turning ended in many a sleepless night, it hit me: do what you did before marriage and kids—real estate.

I told a friend about my new plan. "This will be a great job! I love houses, especially the decorating part, and it'll give me the freedom to come and go for Tim. A lot can happen when a high school student comes home to a vacant house," I reminded her, thinking of my son and the potential parties he might throw if he was left alone on a daily basis. "This'll be easy."

The first big challenge was to pass the real estate exam. When it came to academics, I wasn't the brightest crayon in my parents' Crayola box. What took the average student a day to learn took me weeks. Knowing this would be a craggy mountain I was about to claw and crawl over barefoot, I gave myself five months to prepare.

There were thousands of vocabulary words and definitions to memorize. But what horrified me the most were the math questions. How could I figure out what a client's mortgage might be if I couldn't handle my own checkbook?

If Mr. Smith puts twenty percent down on a home that costs one million dollars, but needs a second loan in the amount of one hundred and fifty thousand, what is the total amount of his first loan? I read the question over ten times with my calculator at my side. I finally put my head down on the table and cried. *Shit, I don't know! I'll never get through this test. I'm just too stupid to ever pass.*

Fortunately, God performed one of His rare miracles and permitted me success in the first sitting. Redoing the test would not be necessary. Soon after, I began to interview with several real estate firms in our town.

In 2004, there were over five thousand agents in Santa Clara County. Realizing "Jackie Madden Haugh" was a nobody among the cast of neighborhood specialists, I thought it best to find a company with an established name and successful track record. Potential clients might not know my name, but Coldwell Banker was universal. It was with this agency that I first hung my license.

I soon discovered the world of a realtor was not as easy as I thought. It was more like being a performer in the mystical show, Cirque du Soleil. You had to be part gymnast and part contortionist, and you needed unadulterated magic to close a deal. Every transaction had its twists and turns, and until the end of the escrow period, nothing was for certain.

At any given moment, a realtor can fall off the high wire she is tiptoeing on and lose the commission that was about to put food on the table for another month. With a traditional job, you can live from paycheck to paycheck. But in real estate, you never know where the next deal will come from, and you're constantly searching for clients.

To begin the arduous task of finding that special person who wants to buy or sell a home, I quickly learned that there were several tricks to my new trade. After six months of intensive training, I sat down at my desk to prepare for my first floor call, a task I had been begging my manager for since my first day on the job.

I thought: *I am so excited! Talking on the phone is my life. How hard can this be?*

My computer was logged in to the Multiple Listing Service. With pen and paper in hand for notes, and a verbal script at my side, I was ready for my first potential client. All I needed was the ding-a-ling of the phone.

"There's a house on Newcastle I want to buy, and I want it today," the high-pitched gentleman's voice on the other end of the receiver informed me.

"Sir, let me check the status of that listing. May I ask your name?" I said, thinking that might be the first piece of information I should have.

"Jerry, Jerry with a J," he snapped, as if I should already have known it due to some telepathic wave traveling through my headset.

"All right, Jerry, *with a J.* It looks like that house is not ready to be put on the market yet. It will be another week before we can get in to see it."

"You don't understand. I want it and I want to buy it today." As he ranted and raged, I could almost feel his hands reaching through the holes of the mouthpiece, encircling my delicate throat like a petulant child who intended to shake me lifeless if he didn't get what he wanted. "I'll give them a good offer and I want them to take it!"

As he proceeded with his tirade, I pictured what he looked like. No doubt he was some wormy little man with beady eyes and a balding head. With short man's complex, the only way he could get anyone to listen to him was to throw a tantrum.

"I am sorry, Jerry, but that's not how things operate here in Los Altos in the current market we're witnessing," I explained, desperately trying to remain calm. "Listing agents and their clients want as many people as possible to see the home. This hopefully will bring multiple offers."

"Well, *that is not the way I operate!*" Jerry-with-a-J screamed into my ear. "If you can't help me, then get me someone who will!" Heavy pounding sounded in the background, which I assumed was his fist on a table. "What is the *matter* with you? Are you new or something?"

"I'm sorry, you're right, *you son of a bitch.* It doesn't sound like we're a good fit," I stated diplomatically. Then I slammed the receiver down. *There is no way I'm referring this asshole to anyone,* I thought. *You're on your own, pal.*

There had to be a better way to snag a buyer. I decided open houses were the way to go. I was good with people face-to-face, and I knew I could make any house sound fabulous with my prolific command of verbal bullshit.

"Jackie, isn't it awful giving up your weekends?" my friends would often inquire. Giving up a weekend was the easy part. It was all the planning and preparation that was necessary before you went through the front door that was so time-consuming.

The worst part of the day was juggling the A-frame signs that shouted out my name at every intersection before I even got to my destination. It would never fail: on any given weekend I was scheduled to hold one of these million dollar beauties open, I'd be thrown a curve ball before I got there.

"Shit!" I yelled at yet another broken heel on my designer shoe. "Why can't this city fix these potholes? This is the fourth pair this month!"

Dressed in my Sunday best (girdle-tight black nylons squeezing in everything I owned and my basic black, ankle-length dress), I imitated Hansel and Gretel, and left my wooden breadcrumb trail to the candy-studded mansion in the hills for its weekend debut. But open houses too would prove to be ineffective, and a big waste of time.

In 2006, eight long, boring, and torturous months had passed in my practice. Not one transaction had been completed or one deal consummated. No paycheck was deposited into my dwindling bank account, and I was broke. Month after agonizing month, I stared at the walls of my office praying the phone would ring.

"Ring, damn it, ring!" I begged anxiously.

Some days life was so quiet in my cubicle that I'd pretend I was talking to a potential client as an associate walked by, just so he wouldn't think I was a loser.

"Excuse me. Please say that again. You want to buy a home for each of your four adult children? No problem."

Even though I doubted I'd ever receive a call, I arrived promptly at nine o'clock dressed in my business clothes, makeup applied to my face with perfection, and hair combed, teased, and sprayed. Once seated at my desk, I began the daily ritual: answering all my personal emails and paying bills. On the surface, I was all business, but underneath, my foundation was crumbling.

And then it happened! The most sought-after creature in the real estate world walked through my door, a referral—that highly coveted client who's been handed to you on a silver platter by a family member or friend. "Hello, Jackie, this is Hung-Su," my friend began on the telephone. "I have a client from China who wants to buy a house here in America. He can spend about five million dollars. Can you help him?"

Five million dollars! I wanted to scream with joy. But, being the trained professional, I politely asked, "When would he like me to show him some property?"

"He'll be in America in a few weeks. Can you start looking for him now?"

I'm ashamed to admit it, but I'm like any other realtor who counts their commission before the deal closes. Thoughts of buying a new car, paying off bills, lending money to the kids, helping the poor, and possibly getting the standard realtor face-lift, ran wildly through my mind. A five-million-dollar sale with a three percent commission meant one hundred and fifty thousand dollars for me. Even though Coldwell Banker would take their split, it would be an enormous amount of money in my bank account. I'd be able to breathe again with a transaction of this magnitude.

Grilling Hung-Su for more information about my soon-to-be "new best friend," I asked about his parameters: what city did he want to live in, and did he want his children to go to public or private schools?

"He knows he wants to live in California, but not sure exactly where," she began. "So let's show him all the high-end areas from Hillsborough to Los Gatos. He needs at least five bedrooms, but would like more because he's expecting to have a maid and a cook. Oh, and he'd like a large yard that has a park-like setting. He needs to meditate daily."

Wow! I need to meditate just to get ready to meet this guy. This is one tall order.

After weeks of nail-biting anticipation, I was to meet Mr. Lee, who had come to America to find a new home. In my black Chevy Tahoe, his entourage all on board, we proceeded. With me acting as the chauffeur, my new client rode shotgun. Hung-Su and Mr. Lee's assistant, Henry, rode in the back. Surveying this motley crew, I couldn't help but be shocked that this multimillionaire, who'd found his fortune at the age of thirty, looked frail, clueless, and desperately in need of a visit from the fashion police. A cigarette hung from the tip of his lip, and his vacant stare led me to believe that quite possibly the synapses in his brain were not connecting.

"By the way, Jackie, Mr. Lee speaks no English," Hung-Su told me.

This should be interesting, I thought.

Once Mr. Lee made the connection that I was the person who would help him find his new home in America, he smiled graciously and bowed his head.

All that was spoken was Mandarin, with a few interjections from Hung-Su for interpretation. The Asian language was bandied about with such velocity, I often wondered if they were arguing. But soon, a giggle would punctuate the dialogue, and I'd know all was right in their world. Back and forth, the words bounced off the interior walls of my car. So, too, went my head turning side-to-side, as I tried to be engaged.

After several minutes of whipping my face back and forth to follow the conversation, I found my mind wandering to all the really important issues in my life: the laundry, paying the endless bills, and doing the dog poop cleanup so the gardener could do his thing without stepping on a million land mines.

"Mr. Lee says he wants a large house with a swimming pool and tennis courts," Hung-Su stated, pulling me back into the job at hand.

"Oh, is he a tennis player?"

"No, he just wants a court to look at. What's that, Mr. Lee?" Hung-Su asked. "He says he also wants enough land for horses. I guess his daughter likes to pet them."

This was getting weirder by the minute. He didn't play tennis, but wanted a court. His daughter didn't ride horses, but liked to pet them. Who *was* this guy?

"Oh, wait, is there a chance we could find all this on a golf course too?"

"Please tell me he at least plays golf," I said.

"No, he just thinks they are pretty. What he really likes to do is work and gamble."

I was beginning to think this meeting was turning into just another lesson in futility. All I really wanted to do was escape to my couch, with my blanket and a bottle of wine so I could drink myself silly. Exhausted and aggravated from listening to the tirade of desires, I tried to be tactful while displaying my expertise as a realtor. But I lost my patience.

"Tell Mr. Lee maybe he should just buy a whole city and then he'd get everything he wants. Plus he could build his own casino!" I stated deadpan, my sometimes-questionable sense of humor raising its ugly head.

Hung-Su giggled as she turned to him to relay the message.

While her tone traveled up and down the musical scale, often ending in the key of high C, I regretted being so flip. *You're so stupid, Jackie. If you are going to stay in this business, you need to learn to deal with all types, even the ridiculous ones with too much money.*

Looking at this gentleman who had only been polite, a little guarded, but polite nonetheless, I wondered: how could I have been so rude?

Slowly, Mr. Lee turned and stared, expressionless, for what felt like my entire lifetime. As he looked me up one side and down the other, I could feel beads of perspiration swell on my neck, and then, drop by drop, traverse down my spine like some ancient method of Chinese torture. Surprisingly, Mr. Lee burst into laughter.

"He said to tell you he likes your sense of humor," Hung-Su conveyed. "He was beginning to think you had no personality, and he hates working with deadbeats." Her face lit up as she continued. "He wants to buy that four-million-dollar home we looked at first."

Oh my God! This is really going to happen. I'm going to sell this home and all my financial troubles for the year are over. I exploded within. I'd be able to pay all my bills, take care of my kids, buy a new car, take a trip to Hawaii, and never lose my nails.

Mr. Lee's limo was scheduled to pick him up in forty-five minutes to transport him to his private jet. Time was of the essence. I needed to get his signature on paper, so with contract and pen in hand we started the negotiations.

"Hung-Su, we need to first discuss his comfort level on price and how long he needs to close the deal."

"Jackie, he will pay full price and all in cash. He only needs three days."

Wow, this just gets better and better. In three days I can go shopping again!

The paperwork began. The lines were filled in, and all the boxes checked. Then my new best friend got a distant look in his eyes and whispered to Hung-Su something that looked serious.

"Jackie, he just realized that he hasn't checked with his immigration lawyer to see if he can bring his children to this country for school next year."

What? Oh my God, stop the presses! The color drained from my face as I thought about what to do next.

Being the moral and ethical woman I am, I smiled faintly. "Tell him there is no point in continuing with this paperwork. The whole reason for buying this home was for his children, and until he knows whether that can happen, he doesn't need a house in America."

Seeing all my dreams momentarily (and monetarily) fly out the window, I held back the tears as I watched the two of them conferring.

"Jackie, Mr. Lee wants to thank you for your patience and honesty. He's used to salespeople trying to force him into a contract and truly admires your integrity."

How special. Yes, I've got integrity, and I'm glad I've earned his respect, but what about my trip! Will I still be able to keep my nails?

Bowing our heads to one another politely while shaking hands, we said our good-byes. I shuffled to my car feeling like I was about to hurl my lunch.

As I drove away, the waterworks from the concrete dam that was holding back my tears gushed forth. My composure crumbled, and sobs heaved from my chest as if I'd just lost my whole world.

But life has an interesting way of putting things back in perspective with just one blink. Walking into my house, I saw my children's smiling faces and was instantly pulled back into my beautiful reality. They were the blessings in my life money couldn't buy.

Did it really matter if we weren't able to take a lavish excursion to Hawaii or buy some hot new wheels or clothes? And how important were my stupid fingernails? Maybe they did make my hands look more attractive, but I could try to grow them naturally. With my artistic ability, I could also learn to paint them myself. What mattered most were the four faces I adored waiting anxiously to see how my day went.

Kissing and hugging each child, I happily announced, "The deal didn't happen today, but let's go out to dinner and celebrate. When do I get you all together in the same place at the same time anymore?"

As with so many times before, I knew I'd somehow figure out how to keep our financial world together. This wasn't the first time in my life things were tight. It was how I'd grown up. Perhaps going back in time was not such a bad thing. I made it just fine then, and I knew I would again.

I think I'll call Dad, I decided as we piled into the car. *Maybe a budget won't be so hard to follow after all.*

Cinderella

It's so amazing how children can rattle cages. When they are little, it's the one they sleep in. When naptime is over, the shaking and crying from their cribs lets the mother know they're done and want out. When they're older, it's the tug of war they pull with the house rules until, once again, the mother lets them off the hook and out the door.

Now it was my cage they were jangling. Only this time, instead of acquiescing to their demands, I wanted to escape to some faraway island where nothing and no one but an occasional tourist could bother me.

Standing in the kitchen with my back against the refrigerator, I felt myself being railroaded into the next phase of my life by my children, whether I liked it or not. I might have given up on the fairy tale of happily ever after, but they hadn't. They were sure my Prince Charming was just around the corner, or at least on the Internet.

Two years after their father left, the kids decided that their mother needed to get back into the land of the living. In their minds, this meant dating. They had forced me out of my cocoon to experience life. Now it was time to find a man to go with the new me. Truth be told, I was sure they were secretly fearful I'd end up an old maid and land on one of their doorsteps in the future.

"Mom, you need to start dating," Michelle said, during a visit home. "It's time!"

"Where in the hell am I going to meet any men? I'm just a mom. What man is going to want me?"

"Oh, poor little Jackie," they all sang at the same time. "Aren't we pathetic?"

"Mom, you're not going to meet anyone sitting on this couch," Jenni announced. "You need to somehow make yourself available for guys to get to know you."

"Yeah, Mom," Lauren chimed in. "I know you don't want to go bar hopping, but there has to be another way to meet nice men. I've heard Internet dating is the wave of the future. You could at least look at some of the sites."

"People are even getting married again after surfing the web," Jenni added.

Great! Now I have to go surfing to get a man. I hate getting my hair wet!

Nevertheless, one evening when the girls were out of the house, I decided to take the plunge. I plopped myself in front of our computer and started searching for Mr. Right with a bottle of wine at my side. I decided if I was going to dive into this new beginning, I'd better be well hydrated. Every site I logged onto promised "true love and devotion or your money back." Being a person who'd try anything once (except illegal substances), I figured I'd bite, but just for this one evening.

I scrolled through the faces of men in my area and desired age range. I couldn't help but think I was sitting at a police station, looking through mug shots of the undesirables life had to offer.

Immediately, I nixed the man covered in tattoos, the gentleman with no hair, and the one with seemingly no teeth. Likewise the jobless freeloaders and those sporting muffin tops (blubber that hangs over the belt line). But the worst had to be the half-naked specimens standing next to their Harley motorcycles.

"Who are these guys?" I mumbled to myself, horrified. "Do they really think any woman wants to look at their hairy chest before she gets to know him? Put a shirt on!"

On the other hand, someone who was educated and could spell when he wrote emails would be wonderful. I knew I was picky in the good-looks department, but they also had to have a functioning brain.

Each gentleman, and I use that term loosely, looked scarier than the last.

Just as I was about to turn off the computer, my fourteen-year-old son walked into the room. "What are you doing, Mom?"

"Hey, Tim, tell me what you think of these guys."

Two seconds later, with a look of deep compassion on his face, he put his hand on my shoulder. "Mom, I'll still love you even if you don't find someone. There has to be some other way. These guys are gross!"

After several hours of painstaking research, I found one face that might work. *Athletic, plays tennis, loves his kids*, or so he said. A man with children was important. He'd be able to understand the complexities of my everyday life and what it took to raise a family.

Bob's profile name was Mr. Giant Guy. He claimed to be six foot four and very handsome. He was looking for a delicate woman with a great sense of humor.

Delicate? That might be a stretch, but people tell me I am funny.

We made contact.

I trudged to my first date in twenty-nine years feeling heavily burdened, as if I were carrying a piano on my back. We were to meet in a restaurant of my choice, far from the beaten track, which I'd picked so no one I knew would see me.

As I looked up and down the street for this mountain of a man, a four-foot-six-inch pipsqueak came up and hugged me.

"You're Bob?" I asked, shocked and confused. "You don't look like your picture."

"Oh, Jackie, I am so happy to meet you!"

"But your profile said you were six foot four."

Rather than towering over my five-foot, five-inch body, his narrow eyes leveled right onto my chest.

"Excuse me, Bob, my face is up here."

"I stretched the truth a little," he replied sheepishly. "Short guys have trouble meeting women, and all the babes are taller."

"What about the picture?"

"Oh, I didn't have one. That's my brother. People say we look alike."

Promising the meal would be on him, he led me into the restaurant.

At least I'll get a free dinner out of this, I thought, realizing I hadn't eaten since breakfast.

Looking across the table at the person I now labeled Mr. Short Guy, I surveyed the physique he'd claimed online he'd gotten from playing tennis. Typically, athletic people have some form and muscular definition. Not this creature. He looked more like the Pillsbury Doughboy than the Michelin Man.

"I thought you said you were athletic."

"Oh, I am. I watch every sports channel I can find," Bob announced proudly.

"What about the tennis you claim you played?" Now I was a little angry, feeling I'd been deceived.

"Table tennis. You know, ping-pong. I'm a champ at that!"

The meal arrived. I shoveled the food into my mouth as fast as I could, hoping to speed up the ordeal. All of a sudden, I felt what I thought was a spider traveling up and down my thigh trying to find its way under my skirt.

"Excuse me!" I shouted.

"I'm a real touchy-feely guy. You don't mind, do you?"

Okay, that does it! "Excuse me, Bob. I have to go to the bathroom." And out the back door I ran.

Several days later I was "winked at" (Internet lingo for "let's get together") by a distinguished-looking gentleman with a manicured beard. In his picture, he was surrounded by his three sons.

"I've been raising my boys, and I'm looking for a good, honest woman to share my life, heart, and home with. I'm Catholic and lead a deeply spiritual life."

This man seemed like a possibility. While his looks didn't reach out and grab me, any man who'd been raising his children all by himself deserved some credit. I hadn't dated a Catholic since college, and even though I was a little wayward, I was deeply spiritual all the same.

The night of our introduction arrived. I drove to the bar and sat in a comfortable lounge chair right next to the emergency exit. I was early. He arrived right on time, with a large bouquet of blood-red roses in hand.

"You must be Jackie," Rich said, lifting my hand to kiss it.

I thought: *Okay, this is creepy. You only give red roses to someone you're passionate about. And who kisses hands anymore? You don't even know if I washed them the last time I went to the bathroom.*

Thirty minutes later, the bright green light that illuminated the exit sign was screaming my name.

"So your bio says you've been raising your sons all by yourself," I said, trying to delve deeper into who this person was.

"I've had my boys the past few years when my ex-wife was out of town on business. Otherwise, she has them full time."

Huh? What is so special about that?

"I'm a deacon at Resurrection Church and I sing in the choir," he added, starting a long dissertation on his dating qualifications. "I attend divorce meetings and I'm the chairman for our singles group, 'Life Without Purpose, Looking for Love.'"

As if all this wasn't sickening enough, he added, "I also run the Bible study sessions and deliver Eucharist to the sick and infirm."

Oh, brother, I'm in big trouble. This man is a religious fanatic.

"So, when can I see you again?" Rich asked, as I downed my glass of wine. "I have a break on Wednesdays between confession and polishing the candlesticks in the rectory. Maybe we could grab a quick bite to eat."

Looking into his soulful eyes, I couldn't help but feel sorry for the guy. How would he ever find a woman who could equal dating the Almighty?

"Rich, I'm sorry, but I don't think there is enough room in your life for me," I said, getting up to make my way out the exit door.

"What?"

"You're already dating someone very special."

From there came a long stream of romantic zeroes: Mr. Freak, the spitting image of the nutty professor from the movie *Back to the Future*, whose long, gray hair danced in the breeze of his windowless station wagon, smoke billowing out the exhaust. Mr. Slimy, the molester with quick, greasy hands who tried to undress me in the parking lot of my favorite restaurant. Mr. Stalker, the pest who called every five minutes. Mr. Mute, the speechless wimp, and Mr. Verbal Diarrhea, the insufferable motor mouth.

Finally, I screamed "uncle" and waved the white flag. Just when I was about to settle back into my favorite spot on my couch, the phone rang. It was my good friend Marsha.

"Would you like to go to a singles lecture and dance?" she asked. "People come from all over the Bay Area."

"What does that mean?" I was afraid this was just another disaster waiting to happen.

"There's a discussion group first, and then they clear the floor for a dance."

"I don't know. I haven't had much success with all this."

"Please come. I promise it'll be fun."

I thought: *I'll try this one last time.*

As I sat in the upstairs party room of an Italian restaurant, I sized up the cast of characters before me. Men and women scattered themselves in the rows of chairs, but all seemed afraid to intermingle as we sat waiting for the speaker.

"I am getting that sick feeling again," I whispered to Marsha.

"Jackie, give it a chance."

"Okay, my gut feelings aren't usually wrong."

A woman wearing clothes that looked as if they came from the "Woman of the Night" section of Goodwill went to the podium and proceeded to promote her new book, *Single and Loving It*. She was loud and unbearable, and to top it off, sweat flew off her body as she flailed her arms while speaking.

"I wish you'd told me to bring my umbrella," I joked to Marsha, ducking the next spray. "Was it necessary to sit in the front row?"

Some of what this woman was saying rang true. No longer did I have to share a king-size bed with a man who snored every night and stole all the covers. My days of acting like a tornado, picking up the house for fear of degrading comments, were over. I was now able to choose when to clean the house (or not) after working all day, raising four kids, and caring for two elderly parents. But to be happy, even *proud*, of being alone because I was dumped for a younger woman? That was a little beyond my comprehension.

"All right, fellow single-ites. It's time you became delighted with your place in life. You need to find the joy that being by yourself brings. You need to dance to the tune of silence," the woman announced, as she gestured to the dance floor. "Thank you for coming. Now go and enjoy meeting all these new friends."

I was definitely not on the same page with extolling the benefits of loneliness. Being a single mom was hard work and often lonely.

"Sorry, but that is one book I plan *not* to buy," I told Marsha, as we put our chairs away. "She probably made herself believe all that crap, since I'm sure no man would get within three feet of her."

The room lights dimmed and the floor cleared for dancing. Looking over my shoulder, I noticed that the bar was a mile deep with people waiting for a dose of liquid courage.

I think I'll join them, I thought as I realized I needed an extra dose of courage too.

As I walked to join them, the DJ turned on his disco ball, and music from the 1970s swirled around the room. To the tune of the Bee Gees' famous hit, "Staying Alive," men began to parade like peacocks, looking for the lucky gals they'd ask to dance. Women strategically placed themselves around the perimeter of the parquet floor, with looks of "pick me, pick me" on their brightly painted faces.

Good choice of songs. That's exactly what I am trying to do, stay alive. I giggled as I noticed the room transform into a sick scene from my youth—the dreaded teen club dance: men on one side, women on the other, and a few couples in the middle.

Nausea rumbled in the pit of my stomach. I quickly found myself running to the far corner of the dance hall where all the other wallflowers waited out the evening. But all was not lost. Standing in the dark, I had a revelation.

On that fateful night, I discovered I no longer cared if I became an old maid. I didn't even care if I died alone. Trying to find a man to date was too much effort. Perhaps "St. Rich" had the right idea. Maybe God was the only partner for me too. I'd heard He was always there for us. Plus, I remembered from my childhood days searching for faith, He rarely talked back. He didn't boss you around and there was no mess to clean up. Yep, maybe the best thing for me to do was become a nun. But first I'd have to do something about those dull black clothes.

Six years later, my prince has yet to find his way to my front door in his shiny BMW to carry me away. I have retired from Internet communication. No more emails from "Sexy Guy, Shy but Handsome," or "Hey Baby, You

Want a Lot of Loving Guy." When I go to bars to have a drink, I go with my girlfriends. I stay away from citywide hook-ups, and if I go to any singles events, it's just to dance and nothing more.

Happily, it wasn't all a waste of time. I was fortunate to meet a few genuine individuals who became dear friends, men who would be in my life forever. With each episode, I traveled a little further on the stepping-stones across the rushing waters of the melting snow of my days, and I found new pieces of me. I learned what I truly wanted and needed in a potential partner: someone who would love me and speak to my soul, not just my body. I refused to settle for less.

Much to my dismay, however, I also discovered I wasn't always the "little miss nicey-nice girl" I'd thought I was. I've been critical, even cruel, with my comments when experiencing new dating opportunities. I even used a few men for companionship, knowing they cared more than I did, to act as filler while I waited for my new life to unfold.

But through it all, the main thing I learned was that I'm a strong and capable woman who can, and will, survive quite nicely on her own. The passion I felt for life and the people who complemented it taught me that I do have something special to offer in the right relationship.

The sweaty writer did have one thing right: You need to know, love, and accept yourself before you can let anyone into your private world. That takes time. That takes patience. That takes perseverance. It also takes a lot of painful honesty.

I'm happy to say that my children no longer worry that I'll end up an old maid. Whether I find Mr. Wonderful or not, for the first time in their lives (and mine), they know I'm happy with whom I've become. They say they love the new me and are proud to claim me as their mother.

It's true. I'm not getting any younger. The mirror shows me that every morning. But all the same, my reflection reminds me of the old Virginia Slims cigarette commercial that stated: "You've come a long way, baby!" And there's still so far to go.

Midge

For most of my young life, I wanted to be just like Barbie, the eleven-inch plastic glamour girl created by Mattel in 1959. I immediately identified with her because I lived with her human incarnation. It wasn't until years later that I discovered Ruth Handler designed the toy after her daughter, not my mother.

"Mom, I want one of those dolls," I screeched every time the commercial played on our black-and-white TV. "She's so beautiful!"

With my face three feet from the television set, I began to sing along with the jingle, "Barbie, you're beautiful. You make me feel my Barbie doll is really real . . . Someday I'm gonna look exactly like you, till then I know just what I'll do. I'll make believe I'm you."

My mom held back her laughter as she watched my head bounce up and down while I sang the ditty, ponytails flying in every direction. "Well, she's very expensive. How much do you have in your piggy bank?"

"The TV says she's three dollars! I have five!" I giggled, dancing in circles. "Can we go to the store right now?"

Few women in our suburban town of San Carlos were ready for their daughters to be playing with such a voluptuous symbol of womanhood. A doll with breasts was unheard of, particularly a doll with large breasts. But my mom saw value in this new creature. Recognizing fashion sense and knowing how to dress with the right accessories was knowledge every little girl needed, especially a plump, awkward kid with sloppy posture and no one but brothers to show her the way.

"Okay, honey. We can go to the store now. I have a few extra minutes to spare."

"You really mean it? Laura's mommy won't let her buy one. She says they're evil or something. What does that mean?"

"Don't worry about what Laura's mom says."

"But she said any mother that allowed her daughter to buy one should be crucified."

For a brief moment, my mother looked perturbed, but quickly changed the look on her face to one of defiance. "She doesn't know what she's talking about. She's just being silly."

As I stood at the counter with my new doll held tightly in my chubby hands, my mom bent over and put her arm around my shoulder. "Now you'll have to save your money. She can't live in a bathing suit her whole life." She kissed my forehead.

I plunked the three dollars on the counter in nickels, dimes, and quarters. "She's going to need some other clothes too."

Rubbing my fingers along Barbie's thin, hard plastic legs and over her torso, I was surprised to feel how firm her breasts were. They were the size of two glass marbles, perfectly perched and always staying in place.

I hope mine will be like this one day. I hate how Mommy's wiggle when she runs.

Earning money became my mission. I wanted my new friend to have every outfit Mattel made for her. When I couldn't find spare change hidden in the cushions of the couch or other living room chairs, I'd crawl on my stomach and search under my parents' bed. If that came up empty, I finally resorted to manual labor and offered to do my brothers' chores, as well as my own.

"Hey Davey, can I take out the trash for you?" I inquired on Saturday mornings. We each received ten cents a week for duties performed around the house.

"Sure, but you have to make my bed too."

"You don't get an allowance for that. That's something we just have to do," I bellowed, feeling completely taken advantage of.

"If you want my allowance, then you have to do other things for me too." Dave smiled, knowing he had me right where he wanted me.

My favorite outfit from Barbie's entire collection was the short ballerina tutu, complete with pink plastic toe shoes that laced up her long legs. As I carefully zipped my doll into the silver sequin bodice and white tulle skirt, I envisioned my mother dancing on a stage, twirling and leaping with confidence as a packed audience clapped enthusiastically. No matter what my mother did, she did it with precision as well as grace.

When I was a child, my mom was the most stunning creature I'd ever seen. Unfortunately, I grew up knowing I'd never look anything like her. Family photos of my father when he was a young boy confirmed that. Except for my ponytails, I was a dead ringer for my namesake; Jack and Jackie looked identical in baby pictures.

Nonetheless, I tried to recreate Mom's image by smearing my face with her lipstick, wearing gigantic earrings, and stomping around the house in her high-heeled shoes.

But what I wanted most was just to be in my mother's striking presence. Unfortunately, she seemed too busy for her only daughter in the early years. There was a house to run, a garden to keep lush, bills to pay, and three overly active boys to keep out of harm's way.

"Jackie, be a good girl and go play with your dolls," she'd say as she gently nudged me toward my room. "I don't have time for you right now."

When Barbie showed up at last, I finally had an opportunity to pretend I was spending time with my mother. This powerhouse of a toy, no taller than a ruler, commanded a huge presence in my nursery of baby dolls. She was long, lean, and self-assured in her business suit, gloves, matching shoes, and purse. She was breathtakingly beautiful in the floor-length glittery black cocktail dress, accentuated with a white fur wrap across her shoulders, and just as glamorous in her zebra-striped bathing suit and hoop earrings, thick, black eyeliner, and ruby-red lips. Barbie had style, grace, and a body right out of *Vogue* magazine. She was an echo of my mother.

My mother, Lassie Pearce Madden, was larger than life itself. In our post-World War II community, every other kid's mother wore a frumpy housedress and had pink sponge curlers in her hair all day long. But Lassie always found a way to look like a million bucks.

"Mom, hurry up," I cried, wanting to get to my friend's house as quickly as possible. In second grade, there were few opportunities for me to play somewhere other than my own home, and I needed to get there fast.

"Honey, a lady never leaves her house without her face on. I'll be right there."

As Mom applied her favorite shade of red lipstick to her voluptuous mouth, and ran a swift brush through her thick, curly red hair, she was finally ready for her day and looking spectacular.

Eventually, the Mattel Company introduced a friend for Barbie named Midge. She was completely unsophisticated, with big blue eyes and freckles all over her nose. Even though Midge wore the same size zero outfits as her predecessor, she never looked quite the same.

I identified with this shy, mediocre creature that seemed to hide in Barbie's shadow. I instinctively knew I'd never measure up to my mom's sophistication but, like Midge, I was grateful just to be in her presence occasionally.

"Hi, Barbie," my Midge doll would say, as I held them face-to-face in my Barbie Dream House. "Want to hang out with me today?"

"Sure, Midge," Barbie responded, dressed to kill in her nurse outfit and cap. "But I can only give you about a half hour. I'm a very busy woman, you know."

I made Barbie saunter to her orange and teal roadster, and then carefully placed her in the bucket seat. With a quick shove, the car rolled out of my room and far away from Midge. Quietly returning to my clone, I sat my blond friend down on the couch of the dollhouse living room to wait for Barbie's return.

"Don't worry, Midge," I whispered, feeling her pain. "I won't make you wait too long."

Fortunately, an evolution began in the Madden household that freed up my mother. My brothers were becoming somewhat self-sufficient. At least they were out of the woods as far as one of them killing the others was concerned. This opened up the possibility for some mother-daughter bonding as time together became more prevalent.

In every generation, during the teen years, daughters typically find their mothers to be the most annoying, ignorant, and out-of-touch human beings on the planet. Not me. At fifteen, I knew I'd never look like my mom. But I thought if I acted like her and held her opinions, I could become just like her. In this new phase of our lives, I was finally given an opportunity to hang out with her. I latched on to each and every moment, afraid that if I blinked, it would all go away.

"Mom, do you want to go shopping?" I asked every weekend, as the men in our lives planted themselves in front of the only television in the house, ready to be consumed by the sporting event of the day. This became our weekly Sunday ritual.

Walking through our usual first stop, Nordstrom in the Stanford Shopping Center, my mother was drawn to a rack in the center of the teen section. "Oh, honey, look at these cute sweaters," she said, pulling two off the rack. "Here, you try the brown one on, and I'll try the green one."

Off we went into the dressing room.

"It looks better on you," I said, watching her turn her glamorous body in circles before the mirror. "You should get it."

"I think we should both get them," Mom announced gaily, smiling at the thought of us looking more like sisters than mother and daughter.

As we stood side-by-side, I couldn't get over the disparity in our physical appearance. She personified a runway supermodel: tall, stately, and stacked. I looked like a stuffed mushroom: short, squatty, and plump at the middle. But, knowing it would make her happy, I concurred and bought yet another garment that would find its way to the bottom of my dresser drawer.

"Okay, Mom, let's do it."

In my high school days, my mom won the attention of all my friends, both male and female. With her charismatic wit and gift for storytelling, she held court whenever someone came to see me.

How does she do it? I wondered sadly, watching my friends become mesmerized. *I wish I could get that kind of attention.*

Throughout those teen years, we were inseparable. I often prayed that some of Mom's social skills would rub off on me, if by no other way than by osmosis. If I could be just a fraction of the woman she was, I'd have it made. I'd be considered smart, competent, and a human magnet, especially to the opposite sex. But low self-esteem and an exaggerated sense of inadequacy kept me from seeing this come to fruition. I knew there was no way this wilted petunia could ever bloom into a magnificent rose. What I didn't realize was that all beautiful growing things one day wither and die.

In the late 1970s, the aging process began to take its toll on Lassie's Barbie-like facade. First came the cancer that carved off her magnificent chest, leaving her maimed and scarred. Next, arthritis eroded the cartilage in both of her hip sockets, causing searing pain. Menopause wreaked havoc with her emotions, and gravity pulled every inch of her once-alluring face south.

Reminiscent of how one of my Barbie dolls looked after she accidentally fell into a campfire, plastic dripping off her smooth face, my mom's skin also began to sag and droop. It was getting harder and harder for her to keep her "face" on with all the fissures traversing the delicate tissue around her eyes and lips. I began to struggle to remember what she'd looked like in my youth. Apparently, she did too.

"Mom, what are you doing?" I asked, catching her looking in the mirror, pulling sagging skin on her chin and neck backward.

Startled, she jumped away from the mirror and began fluffing the pillows on her unmade bed. "Nothing, why do you ask?"

"Why are you holding your face?"

As she turned away, I could see she was about to break down in tears. "If you must know, I was wondering what it would be like to have a face-lift."

"Do you want one?" I knew the answer would be yes if she were to be totally honest, but with her being ever so financially practical, I wasn't surprised at her response.

"No, I'm just trying to remember how I used to look," she replied faintly, a wistful look in her eyes. "I hate getting old."

"Mom, you look great," I tried to reassure her.

She glared and said, with irritation in her voice, "What do *you* know? You're still young."

As the degeneration of her body progressed, so did Mom's self-esteem and confidence. Years of living in pain took away the joy she'd once felt in her life. It seemed all that was left was time to lament: over her failing health, her body, and her parenting skills.

I often found her sitting on the living room couch, staring out to the vacant lot across the street. She talked about all the mistakes she'd possibly made where her children were concerned. She was well into her seventies and gradually putting things in order. The need to fix past blunders became her primary focus.

"Was I a good mother?" she asked one afternoon.

"Why do you ask?" I was perplexed that she would even ask that.

"I want to know if you felt I did things right by you and the boys," she cried, tears bathing her wrinkled face.

"You were the best mother in the world," I reassured, pulling her into my arms. "I don't know where this is coming from."

But the truth was, I did know. It came from that dark place where we all brood from time to time: the place where we question our own worth and value to those we love. It soon became clear that the strong, passionate, and know-it-all exterior my mother had portrayed in my youth was a pretense. She dealt with the same demons I did. We were more alike than I realized, woven from the same delicate yarn.

"I just want to know that I did a good job," she sobbed.

Soon Mom's entire body rejected her. Rheumatoid arthritis invaded not just her hips, but every joint. Spinal stenosis crushed her spine and pinched each nerve into a vise. Walking became an excruciating task. Massive doses of narcotic drugs clouded her once-sharp and stimulated mind, leaving me wondering: *Where did my mom go?*

"Jackie, how old are you now?" she queried one afternoon. She was lying in her bed, surrounded by her pharmaceutical arsenal.

"I'm fifty, Mom."

"*Fifty!* When did *that* happen? How old is Tim?"

"Forty-eight, and Dave is fifty-two."

"Wait, say that again."

"Mom! David's fifty-two, I'm fifty, Tim's forty-eight, and Michael's forty-four." After repeating our chronological order several times, I asked in frustration, "Mom, do you want me to write it down?"

"Yes. I don't know why I can't remember."

Me neither! How could any mother forget the simplest things about her children?

The biggest indignity of all came when her intestines prolapsed and literally fell out of her body. Barbie now needed diapers and her daughter to get through her days. Paying for any health care other than a doctor was unheard of, and she could no longer make it on her own. Midge stepped in to the rescue, now wearing Barbie's nurse outfit.

"Jackie, quick! Come here!"

"I'm coming, Mom. What is it?" I called, racing down the hall to her bedroom.

In less than an hour, I washed the soiled sheets from the night before, cleaned and dressed my mother, picked up the house, and fed my father.

My mother's voice called out: "I'm so sorry. I've had another accident."

Fuck! Not again.

"Okay, let me get some new sheets," I told her patiently, but angrily held back my own tears.

"I'm so humiliated," she sobbed, covering her face with her tattered robe.

"Mom, it's okay. I'll take care of you." Wrapping her up in the one clean blanket left, I led her to the living room. "I won't leave you."

Inside, though, I wondered if I could survive the burden of caring for my disabled mother. At that time in 2003, my life was a disaster. Every step I took seemed to lead to another volcanic eruption.

Like a first-time driver who finally gets her license after three failed attempts, and then smashes into another car on the way out of the DMV, I felt that God wouldn't cut me a break to save my soul. As a result of my divorce, my own heart and self-worth felt like raw meat being shredded through a grinder. The kids were angry and not talking to their father. I had no idea how I was going to pay all my bills, and my mother was dying. I was stressed to the max, with nothing left to give. Like a toy Stretch Armstrong, my limbs were being pulled three times their original length.

"Mom, I'm sorry, but I can't stay very long," I said one day, entering her room to kiss her good-bye.

"What do you mean, you can't stay? I need you."

"I know, Mom, but I have to get back for the kids." I fluffed her pillow, made sure she had her medications, and picked the soiled linens off the floor. "I promised I'd spend time with them today. They have the afternoon off."

"Okay," she replied sadly, looking down to her hands as she played with the sheets. Guilt stabbed me in the heart. "Do what you need to do."

What I needed to do was get on a plane and fly as far away as possible, by myself. But just when I thought I was headed for a nervous breakdown, the hands on the clock of time moved again. The end was near and I had to prepare everyone, including myself, for the inescapable fact: the most important person in my life was leaving.

"Jackie, I'm so sorry, but your mom is very sick this time," her doctor whispered, as we stood in the doorway to her hospital room. "She probably has only about twenty-four hours to live."

"Oh my God!" I blurted. "Are you sure?"

"Yes. The intestines have poisoned her body. She's septic," he tried to explain. "You need to get your father and brothers here."

In a haze, I slowly returned to Mom's side. Looking at this emaciated woman rocking in pain, eyes rolling to the back of her head, I couldn't help but think: *This pathetic creature is not my mother.*

"Mom, the doctor says you are very sick this time," I whispered, leaning in to kiss her cheek.

"Am I going to die?" she demanded, staring straight through me.

Oh God! How do I respond to that?

As I took hold of the same fragile hand I'd held so many other times in tense moments in her life, I quietly said, "I'm sorry, Mom. You're really sick this time."

Before I left to break the bad news to her husband of over fifty years, I waited for the drugs that would take her away to a prescribed coma-like state to kick in. Softly stroking her red hair away from her face, I noticed two months of gray roots sprouting from her scalp. Even in the worst of times, my mother had always looked fabulous. I'd always assumed her red hair was the natural color.

It's nice to know you have your bad hair days too! I thought, as I realized how truly human she was.

Lassie's twenty-four hours turned into six days. As with everything else in her life, she died her way. There was no going peacefully or softly into the night for her. She was going to hang on to every last second, every last laborious breath. My brothers and I took turns sitting by her side, determined she would not leave this world alone.

"Mom, you take all the time you need to leave," I whispered into her ear, crawling into the hospital bed to wrap her in my arms. Cradling her shrunken body, I was reminded how immensely proud I was of her. She was the keeper of all my secrets. Unlike my friends who'd stabbed me in the back, my mom had always had my best interests at heart, and always unconditionally. Now it was time I had hers.

On her last day, the entire family was by her side. The five people who loved her most in the world crowded the tiny, sterile room. Looking at the tubes spiraling out of her arms, monitoring her heartbeat, her every breath, I longed for the woman she once was.

"What is that noise?" I asked the nurse, as gurgling erupted from my mother's throat.

"That's a death rattle," the nurse explained. "She'll probably make several of those before she dies."

As I held my mother's hand for the very last time, she let out one last strong murmur, and then there was silence. Her hand went limp. The process that felt like it was taking an eternity finally ended as she slipped away forever.

"Is she gone?" David asked.

"I think so."

Once the nurse confirmed it, I sat for a moment, paralyzed. What was I going to do without my mother? Who would I ever be able to trust as much as her?

I leaned over and gave her one last kiss. Then I stood up and walked to the door.

"You're leaving?" my father asked, surprised.

"I have to go to the grocery store."

"What? Don't you think you should stay?"

"No. It's time I went home. My children need me."

I couldn't stay any longer. I'd done my grieving long before, while my mom was alive. I wanted to commit to memory the healthy, vibrant woman I'd known as a child; the woman with the infectious laugh who loved to dance around the house as she got her work done; the woman who could turn the simplest story into a chapter from a suspense novel; the selfless person who gave to others but never asked for anything in return.

I thought about how my relationship with my mother had evolved over time. When I was young, she stood beside me, guiding me to the light she felt I must follow. As she got older, I emerged from the darkness. In my light, I was able to see her for who she truly was: a flawed human being like the rest of us. Her weaknesses were intertwined with her goodness and strengths. Like all of us, she was just another child of God making her way through life.

On the outside, my mom was a lovely bronze vase, solid and strong. But she eroded on the inside when personal worth came into question. I, on the other hand, was not the fragile Ming vase I'd always thought I was. It would take a lot more than an earthquake to break me. I was just as strong as any metal, but the big difference between my mother and me was that when I failed, hurt someone, or felt lost, I admitted it. Showing weakness had never been Mom's strong suit.

Walking to my car, I stopped for a second. I couldn't shake the memory of how Barbie had been the personification of my mother. The commercial replayed over and over in my head while I saw my younger self struggling in my role as Midge, the shy and unassuming playmate constantly lingering in Barbie's shadow.

My childhood had been lived in a fantasy world where I manipulated my playthings to suit my needs. Now that I was all grown up, it was time to put away the toys for safekeeping. In my mind, I carefully dressed Barbie in her black-and-white zebra-striped bathing suit and placed her in her cardboard box.

As for Midge, I left her out on display in my room as a reminder of how far I'd come. Only now, she'd be the one wearing that fabulous tutu.

Daddy's Little Girl

"Daddy, please can I go?" I begged relentlessly, as my father got the tackle boxes ready for another fishing excursion with David and Tim.

John Joseph Madden was a gorgeous, six-foot-tall man who looked dashing in business suits as he left for work in San Francisco each morning. Like an older version of Barbie's boyfriend, Ken, he had salt-and-pepper hair that was always perfectly combed in place. He blanketed himself in a quiet demeanor. He had an air of sophistication, something I never saw on any of the other fathers in our small town. But those few times he allowed himself some fun with his children, his kind and gentle manner made my heart melt.

"Jackie, I don't have a rod for you. Be a good little girl and stay home. Your mother needs help with Michael."

"I don't care! I want to come," I demanded, stomping my foot.

Knowing he'd better consent or have a whiny daughter on his hands for days, Dad finally allowed me to tag along to Half Moon Bay.

With my scarred seven-year-old legs dangling over the edge of the rickety Pescadero pier, I held my makeshift rod: a long stick with a nylon string and nail attached at the end. The cold, salty air stung my nose as I watched a parade of seagulls swoop in and out of the murky ocean before me. Dipping the rod into the water, I teased the crabs buried under the rocks, hoping for a bite.

"Do you think I'll catch something?" I asked, anxious to show I had what it took to act like a man.

"Honey, you need to put some bait on the nail." Dad handed me a piece of bacon from the lunch bag and guided the stick directly above the crab's favorite hangout. "Maybe they'll nibble at this." My father got up from his knees, patted my ponytails, and went back to the real task at hand—landing a fish.

A few feet away, the men in my life stood with their gear and tackle boxes. They were busy casting their lines in and out, impatiently waiting for that big bite. I was content to sit alone and wait. The truth was, I didn't care if I caught anything. Just being there, included in the moment, was catch enough. Hours of incessant pestering finally paid off. In that special place in time on that blustery morning, I was one of the boys.

As a child, I craved my dad's attention. Unlike fathers of today, who are both physically and emotionally involved with raising their children, men in the 1950s were solely expected to work and provide financially. Daily interaction wasn't part of the role.

By 1959, we were a family of six. Michael was a baby, and I was entering first grade. My parents' generation rarely got outside help when it came to daily chores, such as gardening, window washing, and house cleaning. They did everything themselves. With all the worries that come with financially supporting a large family, plus the work it takes to run a household smoothly, my dad was on overload. It was no wonder he rarely had time to play, but when he did, it was spent with my brothers.

But, if I ever had any doubt that my father loved me as much as the others, it was erased Christmas, 1960.

Holidays in our house were magical. On that special day, December 25th, it was as if Santa's sleigh ran into a telephone pole, tipped over, and dumped the entire sled down our chimney and onto our living room floor.

My mother didn't believe in wrapping presents. Watching her children dash into the living room and seeing the shock value of an FAO Schwarz replica was her biggest thrill.

Running to my designated section under the tree, I found the usual lineup of dolls, arts and craft kits, and clothes. Then my eyes settled in the corner. Resting on the multicolored, floral wingback chair was a miniature fishing pole and pink tackle box.

"Is that mine?" I screamed.

"Santa brought you your own so you could go fishing with your dad," Mom said, with a special holiday glint in her eyes.

I knew there was no Santa, thanks to one of Dave's friends who'd felt the need to tell me this deflating information a month prior. So I knew there was only one person who could have picked out such a fabulous gift.

"Thank you, Daddy," I whispered in his ear, giving him a tight hug. "It's my most favorite present of all."

In that moment of bliss, I had no doubt, nor ever would again, that he loved me just as much as he loved his sons.

Sadly, however, as the years progressed, he seemed to get busier and busier as I vanished to my room, waiting to grow up. Other than the father-daughter dances in high school, which I treasured, the extent of our interaction was his head popping into my room at night asking if I needed any help with my math homework. My dad and I just stopped doing things altogether. I never questioned his love, but I began to wonder if I really knew this man at all.

It was 1970, and I was about to enter my senior year of high school. Soon I would be out of the house and in college. I knew this was my chance, maybe my only chance, to learn about the first man who'd really loved me. Sadly, I had no idea what made him tick.

"I want you to talk to me," I stated boldly one hot summer night, as we were having dinner together on our patio.

Dad was just about to shovel another forkful of food into his mouth.

He looked up at me. His face became immobile, that recognizable freeze-frame pause when you know something invasive is about to happen.

"Excuse me?" He must have known he was about to be interrogated and that his warm dinner would have to wait, because he reluctantly put the utensil down.

"I want to know what it was like when you were young," I said, with my elbows on the table, my face firmly cradled in my hands.

"Do we have to do this now? Can't I finish my food?"

"We have to do it now. If your dinner gets cold, I'll throw it in the microwave."

My mother was away for two weeks. She had been given the unheard-of opportunity to escape her daily routine and travel to Hawaii on an all-expenses-paid trip with my grandmother. I was put in charge of caring for Dad. The most important task was preparing dinner and serving it promptly at six o'clock. So there we sat, Jack and his daughter, Jackie, all alone with no interruptions.

"I know nothing about your life," I continued. "What was it like when you were a kid? We hear about Mom's life all the time. Was the Depression the same for you?"

Dad looked longingly at his uneaten dinner, let out an exasperated sigh, and answered, "What do you want to know?"

"Well, Mom loves to talk about how difficult it was during the 1930s. She makes it sound as if there were days when people had nothing to eat, and everyone walked around with holes in the bottom of their shoes."

Dad slowly began his tale.

"It was very hard, honey. My father was out of work and we had no money coming in. But even before that time, things were rough. I had a job from the time I was five." As he twirled his fork through his noodles, a wistful expression blanketed his face. "When I was little, I'd help the old ladies in the neighborhood with odd jobs and bring those few pennies home to my parents."

"You were five? What kind of work can a five-year-old do?" In my mind, I pictured the little boy I'd seen in family photos, with curly blond hair and the face of an angel.

"I would sweep floors, pick up groceries at the local market, anything the old ladies couldn't handle." He sat back in his chair. "As I got older, there were the paper routes and helping my dad with his carpentry business. We were broke, but everyone was then, so we did the best we could." Slowly folding the napkin in his lap, he continued, "I don't like to dwell on the bad things in life. If you wait long enough, they change."

Listening to his every word, I was struck with how similar the two of us were. I always knew I looked like his side of his family, but hearing about his positive attitude and approach to life, I realized I was a lot more like him in those ways as well. Being the eternal optimist, I too wanted to believe something good would happen out of any bad situation. Just like my father, I rarely talked about anything that was important to me, either.

"Dad, why haven't you talked about your childhood before?"

"You never asked."

Is that why I've never spoken up? I wondered. *Is that what I'm waiting for, someone to ask me?*

We lingered on the backyard patio for hours. On that warm evening, I grew to know Jack Madden as a father and a man of integrity. My dad was a dreamer, but not for himself. He dreamed of a better life for his children and was determined to do everything in his power to make it happen. He was brilliant and a consummate observer. I remembered how he'd stood on the sidelines, watching his children's every move. My dad had always had a look of pride as he'd smiled from ear to ear, nodding his head in approval.

"Dad, how come you never played golf with your friends?"

"I thought about it, but I had so little time with you children. I didn't want to be away that long on a weekend."

He leaned back in his chair, looking at the stars that were beginning to peek through the dark sky. "On weekdays, I left the house before any of you were awake, and when I got home, you were soon off to bed. I was already missing too much."

In my youth, I wondered if fathers ever felt badly about not being with their children more. Women seemed to have the better gig. Not only could they take their time with household projects and stay in their sweats all day long, but they received the bulk of their children's attention. Now I wondered if my father felt jealous.

"Dad, do you wish you could have stayed home with us and have Mom be the breadwinner instead?"

A loud chuckle rumbled in this throat. Bending forward, he took hold of my hands and confessed, "I think every father wishes that, but that was not a part of what our generation did."

As I got up from the table to take his dishes to the sink, he kissed me on the head, and said, "I thank God every day for what I've been given. To wish or ask for more would be a sin. I'm a truly blessed man."

As the years passed, our relationship grew stronger and closer. I knew that when I went to my mom with a problem or issue, with her powerful and insightful wisdom, she'd tell me exactly what to do. My dad always began with, "What do you want to do? Follow your heart."

When I told my parents I wanted to marry Dave, their reactions couldn't have been more different. My father sat quietly in his red leather easy chair, listening to my every word, as my mom asked in earnest, "Jackie, are you sure you want to do this?"

"Honey, do you love him?" my father asked.

"Yes, Dad, I do."

"Then you have my blessing."

I don't know whether my father really approved or not. I imagine he felt the same as everyone else, but he never said a word against my choice.

On the day he took my hand and placed it in Dave's at the altar, with tears in his eyes, he kissed me on the cheek and turned to my soon-to-be husband. "Please promise me you'll take good care of her."

One minute I was his little girl, the next, I belonged to another.

As my babies came into the world, I could see my parents travel back in time to my own childhood.

"I'll never forget the day you were born," Dad began, as he gently stroked the hand of his first grandchild, Michelle. "You were the most beautiful creature I'd ever seen. I fell in love with you immediately."

"Do you want to hold her, Dad?" I asked, watching him look longingly at the plump bundle swathed in a soft, pink blanket.

"Can I?"

My mother got out of the chair so my father could take a seat and carefully placed my baby in his loving arms.

"Now, Jack, be careful of her head."

"I know, Lassie."

"Don't hold her too tight."

"I know, Lassie."

I studied him as he embraced my baby girl. My imagination placed me in those strong arms twenty-eight years before. *I bet that was the same scene in my hospital room.*

"Make sure her face isn't covered with the blanket. She needs to breathe."

Looking up at his wife, trying to contain his frustration from her barrage of orders, Dad simply said: "I've done this before."

As another link in the chain of the Madden family lineage appeared, my dad was able to be the openly loving person he was too busy to be when my brothers and I were young.

"Your father is driving me crazy with all his questions," my mom said angrily, as she arrived for her weekly visit and cup of Folgers instant Café Vienna coffee. "Every time I get home, all I hear is: What are they doing? Did the babies say anything new and are their bowel movements regular?" She swirled her coffee and stared at the creamy concoction that now resembled a whirlpool ready to suck her in. "He is driving me crazy! What man cares about a poopy diaper?"

"Mom, I think he's just enjoying watching them grow."

"Well, you're my daughter and I care what happens to *you*. Does he ask you questions about your life? No!"

Going back to my lukewarm mug, I thought about why my mom was so angry. Michelle enjoyed the gift of the man my mother always wanted for me when I was little. Mom was angry, maybe even envious, at what she felt we'd missed. But I couldn't be angry. I already knew he loved me. Now I had the joy of watching my father's love for my children.

In an effort to calm my frustrated mother, I covered her tense, arthritic fingers with my hand. "Mom, I know how hard it was to raise us. You felt completely alone sometimes."

Her outburst was like so many others: the result of dark, murky waters running deep, weaving past the days gone by.

"I understand that you wish Dad had been there to help you more, but I love seeing him with my kids. He now gets to be the father he always wanted to be."

Twenty-five years later, the roles of my parents and myself had reversed, putting me in place as part of the "sandwich generation." I felt like a piece of bologna smashed between spicy mustard and moldy, limp lettuce. On one side, I was raising overly spirited, cantankerous, foul-mouthed teenagers. On the other side, I was caring for my crippled, elderly parents.

As far back as I could remember, my parents had both stated they never wanted to be a burden. They'd told me over and over: "Just put me in a home." But the truth is that no one wants to be shut away, especially my father. He worked so hard all his life, and he deserved to live the twilight years the way he wanted.

After my mom died, my attention drifted to him. His body became his biggest opponent on the playing field of daily existence. A stroke twenty-four years earlier had caused paralysis in his left arm and left the matching leg nearly destroyed. Now, that limb was totally worthless, and all that still functioned was his right arm. Terrified he'd one day end up in a nursing home, I made a vow.

"Dad, I promise, I'll take care of you," I assured him. I didn't realize those words would become the biggest challenge of my life.

My father wanted things his way, and that meant he'd only allow help for a few hours a day. One day, I found him all by himself.

"Dad, you need more care than this," I stated firmly. "What if there's an emergency? You can't do anything to help yourself."

"There won't be an emergency."

"What if there's a fire or an earthquake?"

"There won't be."

"Dad! We could have an earthquake any day, and your house caught fire once before."

"Jackie, I'm fine. Nothing will happen. What can anyone do for me anyway? I don't want to pay for someone to sit around." He gave me his famous impish, Irish grin. "This is the way I want it."

Fear and frustration kept me awake at night. Knowing my ninety-three-year-old father was in his bed from five o'clock in the afternoon until nine o'clock in the morning each day, with no one close by, caused guilt to invade my every waking hour.

"How about you come live with me?" I asked him.

"That won't work, Jackie."

"Sure, it would. You could have Jenni's room. I can make the bathroom handicap accessible." I started thinking of all the ways I'd have to change my home to include rails, ramps, and bedside urinals.

"I can't do that. You'd drive me crazy!"

I'd drive you crazy? I wanted to scream. How could I be the one to drive this man nuts? I was the loving daughter, the devoted daughter, the child who cleaned up all of life's little messes, including the adult diapers. There was no way I could be the annoying one.

Surveying the home my father had lived in for the past fifty-three years, I noticed our family history in photographs scattered about the living room. In the corner, by his favorite chair, was a mountain of books that he'd read, piled halfway to the ceiling. On every table, my mother had lovingly left behind a decorative item. I wouldn't want to leave the only happy home I'd lived in, either.

But to make sure, I asked one more time: "Dad, you're sure you don't want to live with me?"

"Thank you, Jackie, but no. I like my life the way it is." He smiled sweetly. "Just come visit when you can."

"Okay, but you have to have more than a few more hours of help at home. There's no more discussion about that."

Now when I visit, we go over every detail of each other's lives. We talk politics, sports, and finances. At least, he does, and I sit in amazement at the sharpness of a mind making its way toward one hundred years. My dad is the consummate loving father and teacher, a true inspiration.

No matter how old I get, I'm still that strawberry blond, ponytailed child who followed him from room to room just to be near him. It doesn't matter that I got a college education, successfully worked at several jobs, and held my life together after divorce. To Dad, I'll always be his little girl.

Now, when I'm tucking him into his bed on my regular visits, I lean over and say, "I love you, Daddy." The one strong limb left on his body pulls me to his chest, and he kisses me. Holding back the tears I know will come when I leave, he whispers, "I love you too, honey. You're a good girl."

Dancing Queen

As I walked into the warehouse that cool Saturday evening in June 2007, I was struck by the sheer magnitude of the twenty-foot, floor-to-ceiling metal poles scattered throughout the dimly lit space. This was no ordinary dance hall.

"Shit, I think I'm in trouble," I said, looking at the other participants in the room.

As I watched the other women stretching their long, flexible bodies in preparation for the adventure, I wondered how, in their fifties, they could still pull their feet behind their ears. At fifty-five, I could barely bend over to tie my shoes.

Two scantily clad young women, with their sculpted legs dangling from the hemlines of extremely short shorts, entered the room. Lindsey, a petite but athletic-looking woman with a Betty Boop hairdo, gave the class introduction. Aheisha, a six-foot-tall bohemian beauty with legs that traveled to her throat, paraded around the room in red leather thigh-high boots and a barely-there black lace outfit, demonstrating exotic moves we'd all be expected to replicate.

"Where are the whips and chains?" I whispered to the woman next to me whose face indicated she was in an advanced state of shock.

"Okay, ladies, everyone pick out a pair of shoes and let's get going,"

Lindsey called out, above the giggles masking the trepidation infiltrating the room.

Along one wall, a large rack held six-inch black stiletto heels in every size. Looking at those potentially deadly weapons made my nerves churn. The last time I'd ever worn anything like that was in the 1970s when I was a disco diva, sporting white double-knit bellbottoms and floral print silk blouses. I didn't model them well then, and I was reminded of the old saying: *If it didn't look good on you when you were young, don't try to repeat it when you're old.*

"I'm sure I'm about to break an ankle, if not kill myself," I muttered, squeezing my size eight foot into a size six shoe. "Who ever thought this was a good idea?"

"Yeah, I can't believe I'm doing this either," a voice from behind me whispered, obviously feeling my pain.

But the one thing life had taught me was to be adaptable to any situation, roll with the punches, and be open to new possibilities. Determined to be a good sport at this pole dancing birthday party, I mustered all my strength to survive what I expected to be an evening from hell.

"Laura, do you mind if I hold onto your head while I try to stand?" I asked the woman sitting next to me.

"No, go ahead, just as long as you'll give me your hand when it's my turn to get up."

Sizing up more of my surroundings, I stated, "Let's slide our butts over to that rack of shoes. That'll give us something steady to grab onto."

Scooting our rear ends across the floor, we made it to the wooden frame. By positioning myself just right, I managed to get to my knees, and then gingerly onto each foot. Looking around the room, I was comforted by the fact that the fifteen other women in our group were having just as much trouble navigating themselves to an upright position as I was.

"Ladies, who would like a martini?" a couple of eager participants shouted. "This is a birthday celebration. Drink up!"

"Hmm, drink up? No problem." I snickered. That was one thing I was becoming good at in scary moments, but my choice of poison was typically wine. Martinis had never been a viable libation for me. But in light of the fact that I was about to pole dance, the liquid fire never seemed so appetizing.

Approaching the bar, I picked up the clear drink. As I quickly threw back my head, the first shot went down smoothly.

"Oh my God, Jackie! You're supposed to sip that," Teresa, the birthday girl, explained.

"Can I have another?" I asked sheepishly, knowing I would need several more to loosen up.

"Jackie, relax," Teresa advised, as she handed me my second glass. "You can learn to gyrate just as well as you wiggle. I know you've been dancing your whole life."

I watched her pick out her personal pole, her main squeeze for the evening. She began curling her petite, five-foot-two ballerina body around it like a boa constrictor preparing for a feeding. When the music began, she attacked her movements with a vengeance.

Watching her spin this way and that, thoroughly enjoying the experience, I couldn't help but think back on my youth and what dancing meant to my life. Music had always been my best friend. It allowed me to express every emotion I guarded from the world around me. I could be whoever I needed to be in the confines of my small bedroom, as I moved my body to a rhythm that not only pulsated through me, but spoke to my soul.

After being expelled from dance classes at the age of eight, I'd made up my mind that no matter how difficult a dance move might be, I'd never give up trying to master it. As I stared at the steel rod before me, that age-old determination boiled to the surface, and my will to triumph exploded.

"Ladies, are we ready?" Lindsey called out, strutting across the floor. "Everyone stand and line up against the wall."

One by one, the tipsy revelers got to their feet and teetered over to the mirror, desperately holding on to one another like a line of black-and-white dominoes. We knew that if just one of us faltered, we'd all go down, one right after the other, and land in one large pile of intertwined legs, stilettos flapping in the breeze.

"Jackie, don't let go of me. I don't think I can make it," my friend Mary whispered.

"You can make it. Just hold on tight." We held our backs close to the wall, fear plastered on every waiting face.

"Now, the first thing you have to learn is the walk. You know, that swagger one does when trying to get a man's attention," Aheisha said.

With a twist of her hips, this woman of the pole strategically lifted one leg and then crossed it diagonally over the other. With each provocative step, she landed on the balls of her feet in tiptoe fashion. For extra sex appeal, her fingers combed through her waist-length hair, before she flipped the curly auburn locks from side to side.

"What's with the pout on her face?" I asked Mary. Peering into the mirrored wall, I practiced making contortions with my lips, puckering them vertically and then horizontally.

"Sorry, Jackie. You look more like a blowfish than a seductress."

Realizing she was right, I focused on the lower part of my body to attain the look, first by stroking my hands up and down my thighs and then bending my knees to form the perfect, seductive plié.

Like baying sheep being herded into the slaughterhouse, we followed each other single file, mimicking the instructor's every move.

"I feel like such a dork. Maybe I need longer hair to feel sexy enough for this charade," a woman sighed to my left. "I'm never going to get this. I quit."

Looking at this discouraged individual, I realized she was probably ten years younger than I was. She was exquisite with her long, lean dancer's body, and wrinkle-free face, but was obviously way out of her comfort zone. Her resignation made me that much more unwavering in my desire to take control of the evening.

I'm going to somehow get this or perish in the effort! Just because I'm fifty-five years old doesn't mean I don't have what it takes, I decided as I watched this dejected beauty slither to the sidelines.

With a snap of her three-inch long, candy-apple-red fake fingernails, Aheisha called out: "Find a pole for some tricks. Now the fun begins."

"Oh goodie, I'm ready! Learning tricks is my life," I snickered. "How else did I get those kids to do what I wanted?"

Looking around the room, I noticed sheer terror on all the faces. Carefully, we left the wall and wobbled to a pole that would save us from falling over. Holding on for dear life, I anxiously waited for the lessons that might possibly end my life, or worse, my dignity.

"Mary, please share this pole with me," I called out, laughing over the silliness of it all. "I need someone I trust to feel my pain."

"I'm right there with you, but don't make fun of me."

"Oh, honey, you've got to be kidding. I think that's the whole reason behind this farce." I gave my friend a hug. "You don't think Teresa thought we'd take this seriously, did you?"

"I don't know. Just look at her. She looks like she's been doing this her whole life."

Watching our birthday girl friend work the room, I wondered if Mary wasn't right. Teresa was very comfortable, maybe a little too comfortable, with the evening.

"Do you think she secretly has a pole in her bedroom?" Mary whispered.

"That could be why her husband always has a smile on his face."

In the next hour, we learned to drop and roll around the bar in concentric circles that spun faster and faster, with one leg hanging on, until we finally landed somewhat dizzily on the floor.

Then, there was the backbend straight out of a Barnum & Bailey Circus act, where our hands guided our curved bodies down the post and finally to the ground. Contortionist was never among the list of titles I possessed, but somehow, precariously, I made it.

"Ladies, as the back of your head touches the floor, you can begin to lay your shoulders down and then the rest of your body. But don't forget the sexy kitten pose at the end."

"Help! I'm stuck!" I was mortified, knowing I didn't even come close to anything sexy, especially a kitty. "Someone please untangle me." Looking at Mary, I sneered, "She expects us to *pose*, too? I think I'll just lie here until it's time to go home."

"Quick, Jackie, get up. She's onto another trick."

There was the bump and grind with pelvises thrusting back and forth as we maneuvered around our cold, silent partner, followed by more drop and rolls.

As if all that wasn't enough, we were then told to scale the iron shaft, pulling our bodies up one hand over the other toward the ceiling. With stilettos still securely strapped to the feet, our upper torsos then fell backward, while our legs gripped the bar like the clenched jaws of an animal trap.

With the crowd's nervous giggling resembling the sound of naughtiness being caught in the act of doing something inappropriate, I began to wonder if we'd found a new "joy toy," only one that was a little harder to take to bed. There I was, twelve feet off the ground, both legs crisscrossed around the metal demon, my upper body leaning backward and arms thrashing in the air.

"Hey, look at me! I'm doing it! I'm doing it!" I screamed at the top of my lungs.

I methodically descended back to earth, amid the cheers of my fellow dancers. I was struck with an epiphany. Without realizing it, over the past seven years since my divorce, this little lost girl had undergone a metamorphosis into an empowered woman who wasn't afraid to try anything.

Taking a bow and enjoying my newfound glory, I was hit with the symbolism of what had just transpired. The pole adventure had begun just like any other obstacle that was put in my path. I'd known it would be difficult, but I'd made a conscious decision to overcome it. I've always been a fighter, but in my younger years, I'd taken on the challenges to prove something to everyone else, or to win their love, never for self-satisfaction.

In front of the mirror before me was the reflection of a confident woman who now took on challenges to validate only herself. I'd always envisioned myself as an overfed hippopotamus. As each costume in my life was thrown my way, it seemed I'd had to suck everything in tight in order to stuff my body into it.

Looking into the mirror, I was caught off guard by the strong, lean, regal image in tight black spandex and stiletto heels. More importantly, I was thrilled by the fact that I no longer cared what other people thought.

A family priest had once described me as the girl with liquid steel running through her veins. "Mrs. Madden, as Jackie grows older, that strength will be her saving grace. But she must learn to use it for herself, and not as a tool to impress others."

Nowhere had that prophecy become more apparent than during my divorce. Entering marriage, I'd still had no idea who the real "Jackie" was. Over the years, I'd become even more lost in the maze of rearing children, caring for aging parents, winning my husband's attention, and taking on volunteer work. I'd thought that in being the perennial pleasure provider to others, I'd find fulfillment. What I'd found instead was an exhausted woman, always searching for, but never finding, self-satisfaction.

Being firmly planted under the thumb of an overly confident man who appeared to have all the answers on how everyone's life should operate had made me doubt myself even more. What little confidence I might have had at the beginning of our marriage fizzled through the years, as if I were a balloon slowly dissipating until all that was left was a plastic shell of the bright color it once was.

But when Dave left for another woman, I'd known it was time to stand up for myself, take charge, and be the role model my children needed. Betrayal was not something I'd proclaimed during my wedding vows. Within just a few short weeks of his exodus, I'd filed for divorce.

I hugged my pole that evening, no longer out of fear but out of a sense of victory. This thing that was initially my nemesis was now my friend, an unsuspecting ally that helped me to acknowledge that I'd arrived and was no longer afraid.

As the women congregated in the lobby after the party, I noticed a list of classes on the wall. I grabbed a brochure and ran to the adjacent dance attire shop to purchase the right clothes. "Now I'm ready for round two!" I called out, as I twirled my itty-bitty black micro-mini top. I thought: *The second half of my life is going to be great!*